Crit **ctice**

Critical Reflection in Practice

Generating Knowledge for Care

Second Edition

GARY ROLFE, MELANIE JASPER AND
DAWN FRESHWATER

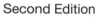

palgrave
macmillan

First edition 2001 (previously entitled *Critical Reflection for Nursing and the Helping Professions*)
Reprinted eleven times
Second edition 2011

Published by
PALGRAVE MACMILLAN

Palgrave Macmillan in the UK is an imprint of Macmillan Publishers Limited, registered in England, company number 785998, of Houndmills, Basingstoke, Hampshire RG21 6XS.

Palgrave Macmillan in the US is a division of St Martin's Press LLC, 175 Fifth Avenue, New York, NY 10010.

Palgrave Macmillan is the global academic imprint of the above companies and has companies and representatives throughout the world.

Palgrave® and Macmillan® are registered trademarks in the United States, the United Kingdom, Europe and other countries.

ISBN 978–0–230–20906–0

This book is printed on paper suitable for recycling and made from fully managed and sustained forest sources. Logging, pulping and manufacturing processes are expected to conform to the environmental regulations of the country of origin.

A catalogue record for this book is available from the British Library.

A catalog record for this book is available from the Library of Congress.

10 9 8 7 6 5 4 3 2 1
20 19 18 17 16 15 14 13 12 11

Printed in China

Contents

CONTENTS

List of figures and tables

Figures

LIST OF FIGURES AND TABLES

Tables

Acknowledgements

The authors and publishers are grateful to the following publishers and organizations for granting permission to reproduce copyright material: Kappa Delta Pi, International Honor Society in Education, for Figure 3.1, originally from Dewey, J., *Experience and Education* (New York: Macmillan, 1938); Wiley-Blackwell Publishers for Table 3.2, originally from Kim, H.S., 'Critical Reflective Inquiry for Knowledge Development in Nursing Practice', *Journal of Advanced Nursing*, 29, 5, pp. 1205–12 (Oxford: Blackwell Science,1999), and for Figure 6.6, originally from Heath, H. and Freshwater, D., 'Clinical Supervision as an Emancipatory Process', *Journal of Advanced Nursing*, 30, 5, pp. 1298–1306 (Oxford: Blackwell Science, 2000); Ashgate Publishing for Figure 7.1, originally from Brown, A, *Groupwork* (Aldershot: Gower Publishing, 1992). Every effort has been made to trace and contact all copyright-holders, but if any have been inadvertently overlooked the publishers will be pleased to make the necessary arrangements at the first opportunity.

Preface

The changing face of professional practice and education

The decade since the publication of the first edition of this book has witnessed unprecedented changes to the ways in which healthcare professions in the UK work to provide care to patients. Factors such as the global economic costs of health care, European working time regulations which affected, in particular, junior doctors' hours, and the growth of professional regulation have all changed the dynamics of practice within which all practitioners work. There has been increasing recognition of the independent roles that experienced practitioners in all fields of health care can play in taking both accountability and responsibility for healthcare assessment, diagnosis, care package planning and delivery, moving many functions from the sphere of medical practice to other recognized professional practitioners. This has resulted in the development of consultant roles in all healthcare professions, and has seen a huge increase in the number of specialist practitioners. The global economic crisis occurring as we were revising this book has resulted in threats of huge reductions to public spending in the coming years, putting extra strain on the UK NHS's already creaking budgetary controls. In short, spending on healthcare has to be reined in.

These developments in the healthcare agenda have been accompanied by changes in the ways that healthcare professionals are trained and educated. Some disciplines such as nursing are now firmly embedded in the university sector, while other emerging professional groups such as paramedics are just beginning to engage with higher education at pre-qualification level. Indeed, a workforce educated at least to degree level is usually regarded as one of the defining features of a profession. Clearly, healthcare practice and healthcare education are essential partners, and neither can flourish without the other.

For example, we have recently witnessed the growth in power and influence of notions of evidence-based practice (EBP) as the key to decision-making in healthcare. The evidence-based practice movement began as an educational initiative, and has built its success on a symbiotic relationship between the universities as promoters of the theoretical ideas which underpin it and as suppliers of evidence for practice, and the healthcare professions who maintain a constant demand for that evidence. However, the rise of EBP in the health professions can also be partly attributed to the type of knowledge that it promotes. Newly emerging professions and academic disciplines often rely heavily on traditional ideas about what constitutes good practice and sound scholarship, and this usually results in a very technical approach to practice based on 'hard' scientific evidence. As a result, EPB is usually regarded as the dominant discourse and the default mode of practice for most healthcare professions.

It is in the face of this growth in technical practice based on hard scientific evidence that we are attempting to justify and promote practice based primarily on reflection on and in our own practice. It is probably fair to say that reflection, both as a way of practicing and as an approach to learning, has forged a somewhat ambivalent relationship both with the emerging healthcare professions and with their developing partnership with higher education. On the one hand, interest in reflection both as a way of learning and as a way of practicing has often emerged at the point at which the professions first begin seriously to address their academic standing. Reflection, then, is promoted by some academics as an innovative learning strategy for exploring professional knowledge. On the other hand, the type of knowledge that serious and critical reflection produces is sometimes seen as directly challenging, and even contradicting, the type of knowledge that is valued most highly in universities and practice areas, which favour those types of knowledge to be found at the top of the hierarchies for evidence-based practice. In fact, the evidence-based paradigm challenges or even dismisses many of the concepts that we believe to be essential for the development of critical reflective practice and the creation of experiential knowledge and theory for practice. We are therefore concerned that the strides that have been taken in raising the profile of independent practitioners and their capacity to provide individualized care based on expertise and experience will be eroded in favour of protocol and procedurally driven care measured against governmental targets which tell us nothing of the experience of patients or the true outcomes of care delivery.

Hence, our motivation in revising this book has been to continue to promote the centrality of critical reflection as key to experienced and expert professional practice. We propose that reflective learning is *the* way of life for committed professional healthcare practitioners who are always striving to give the best and most appropriate possible care. This involves not only the development of an individual knowledge and skills base, but also the growth of confidence to challenge some of the taken-for-granted assumptions endemic in healthcare and the empowerment to champion what is right rather than what is dictated.

The coming of age of reflective practice

As well as structural, political and professional changes in most health and social care disciplines, the past 10 years has also seen the growth and development of reflection as a way of doing practice and education. When we wrote the first edition of this book, reflecting on our own practice was still a relatively novel way of thinking about and learning from what we do as healthcare professionals. Arguably, of course, the notion of reflection can be traced back at least 2,500 years to Socrates' assertion that 'the unexamined life is not worth living', but its modern application to professional learning and practice probably dates from Donald Schön's book *The Reflective Practitioner*, published in 1983.

As with individuals, the growth and development of academic ideas and practices progresses in stages. Seen in this light, reflective practice could be regarded as a somewhat unruly and challenging 18-year-old when we published the first edition of our book in 2001. In the intervening years, that teenager has matured into a thoughtful and (perhaps) rather staid and conforming young adult.

As a rebellious youth searching for its own identity while at the same time challenging the established 'unexamined life' of nursing and healthcare practice, the academic discipline of reflection produced a flurry of publications during the 1990s, including many of the seminal works still being cited today. However, as Thomas Kuhn (1996) pointed out, most scientific revolutions or paradigm shifts are relatively short-lived and are followed by periods of 'normal science' where the shift in focus or perception is consolidated and embedded. That has certainly been the case with reflective practice, where the flood of challenging and radical publications of the 1990s has given way to a steady trickle of more conservative texts which largely restate and establish reflection as a mainstream practice.

These developmental changes have had three implications for our book. First, while we have restructured and largely rewritten the vast majority of the text, many of the seminal references continue to be of relevance and can still be found in the second edition. Reflective practice might have grown up, but it is still very much influenced by its childhood and adolescence. Second, like most young adults, reflective practice has 'left home' and is growing in influence in disciplines and professions across the entire spectrum of health and social care practice and education. For this reason, we have widened our scope and modified the title of our book to *Critical Reflection in Practice*. Third, our target readership has grown up and matured alongside the development of reflective practice. Many of those who might have found the first edition of our book useful in their undergraduate education and early years of professional practice are now senior practitioners who also teach, supervise and mentor their colleagues. While the second edition continues to be of relevance to beginning and novice reflective practitioners, we have made a deliberate effort to ensure that it will also be of use to senior practitioners in health and social care in relation to their own higher education and to the education and development of their colleagues.

Finally, we would like to briefly restate our guiding principle as outlined in the preface of the first edition. As before, we have tried to write a book that is not simply *about* reflection but which employs a reflective methodology. We have therefore retained the three strategies of using real-life case studies to illustrate our points, of encouraging you to take 'reflective moments' to think about your own experiences, and of offering suggestions for further reading. To repeat the claim we made in the first edition, if this book teaches anything, it teaches how you might best learn for yourself.

GARY ROLFE
MELANIE JASPER

1

Critical reflection and the emergence of professional knowledge

Melanie Jasper and Gary Rolfe

Introduction

No one involved in professional practice and education in health and social care could have failed to notice the inexorable rise of evidence-based practice over the past decade. As the health and social care disciplines strive to become accepted as bona fide professions with all that entails, there is a perceived demand for practice to be based on firm evidence and for evidence to be based on good science. Evidence-based practice is therefore often taken to mean *research*-based practice, and research is taken to mean experimental or quasi-experimental empirical studies. In this chapter, we will outline the challenges posed by the knowledge demands of the emerging healthcare professions and examine how these have shaped our thoughts about the need for a critical approach to reflection. We will argue that critical reflection can make an important contribution to the evidence-base for practice, but more importantly, that it can reflexively influence practice in its own right.

More specifically, our aims for this chapter are:

1. to help you to think about the professional constraints and pressures that determine the way you practice;
2. to encourage you to think about the ways in which you reflect on your practice as part of your everyday life;

3. to explore the ways that you might avoid reflecting on difficult or uncomfortable issue; and
4. to begin to think more critically about yourself and your practice.

Reflective moment

Think carefully about our aims for Chapter 1. Now think about your own practice and how these aims might contribute towards developing it. For example, what initial steps might you take in order to become a more critical reflector?

Based on our aims above, identify and write down some of your own aims, both in terms of what you hope to know and what you hope to be able to do after reading Chapter 1. We will return to these at the end of the chapter.

Developing professionalization in healthcare

The past decade has seen changes to ways in which the multitude of health and social care occupations are regulated in the UK, with increasing emphasis on public protection and risk reduction. The three regulatory bodies concerned with all healthcare professionals except medicine, the Health Professions Council (HPC), the Nursing and Midwifery Council (NMC) and the General Social Care Council (GSCC) (the latter with separate bodies for Wales, Scotland and Northern Ireland) were established from their predecessors in 2001, provide far more emphasis on professional accountability and behaviours through codes of conduct, standards and ethics for registrants than previously. All councils are charged with setting standards for entry to a professional register, for approving programmes for education and training, for maintaining a register of practitioners and for taking action against registrants who are not meeting their standards of practice. The Health Professions Council alone now has over 200,000 registrants on its active register, regulating 14 professions in 2009, but with at least four more professions likely to come under its remit in the next five years. In addition, there are moves to incorporate healthcare practices previously considered to be 'alternative' such as acupuncture, medical herbalists and traditional Chinese medicine practitioners. The NMC has around 680,000 registrants.

The scope of activity of the Councils ensures that expanded areas of professional practice are initially regulated in the same ways as entry to the professions. For instance, programmes leading to independent and supplementary prescribing by nurses, midwives, pharmacists, and some other allied health professions such as physiotherapists and radiographers must be approved by the NMC and/or HPC, dependent on the profession involved. A recent exploration of higher levels of practice by the NMC takes the stance that what is regarded by many as advanced practice bears no additional risk to the public than the basic notion of competence to practice, and at that time declined to set standards for advanced practice *per se*. However, a change of leadership at the NMC has resulted in a declared intention to re-open this debate, especially in light of increasing changes to the ways in which doctors work, and the resultant impact on the work of specialist and consultant nurses. The protection of the public is of paramount importance in the work of all the regulatory bodies, and at a time when there is growing criticism of standards of practice within the NHS, it is the responsibility of the professions to ensure that whatever role the practitioner is performing, it is being performed in compliance with the standards and codes of practice expected. Similarly, the HPC has not indicated any intention to consider registration beyond competence to practice on registration. All Councils do set standards for continuing professional development and require evidence of this for periodic re-registration, but this attests only to the standards required by all practitioners and does not differentiate further levels of practice in any way.

Yet, surely, the public must have expectations of practitioners who have been qualified for a long time, or indeed hold titles such as 'Consultant', 'Advanced Nurse Practitioner', or 'Specialist', even if the professional bodies do not. At the very least, every practitioner is expected to ensure that they practice to the latest (and best) evidence available, to keep themselves abreast and skilled in the latest treatments and techniques available and to practice within the Codes of Conduct published by their respective professional bodies. How would a member of the public be able to judge that a practitioner does indeed measure up to their expectations?

Reflective moment

Think about the last time you or one of your family used the services of a registered healthcare practitioner. How did you know that they

3

were competent to practice? What evidence did you have that allowed you to draw that conclusion? What would give you confidence in their professionalism, over and above such things as certificates on the wall, titles, uniforms or name badges?

The increasing professionalization and regulation of healthcare professions is aimed to increase public confidence in them following such cases of professional misconduct as Harold Shipman, Beverley Allitt, the Bristol Paediatric Heart Surgery and retained body parts incidents. The end result is expected to be greater patient safety, but there is no evidence available to demonstrate that this is indeed the case – it is an assumption arising from tighter legislative control. It is, in fact, hard to see how better patient care arises from imposing more regulation on practitioners; indeed, it is the central tenet of this book that better patient care will only result from enabling all practitioners to be critically reflective within their practice environment.

Becoming critical

It is primarily this challenge to find ways of promoting better patient care that prompted us to write a book about what we call critical reflection. In the preface to the first edition to this book we described critical reflection as 'using the reflective process to look systematically and rigorously at our own practice' (Rolfe et al., 2001). We might have added that critical reflection also uses the reflective process reflexively to look systematically and rigorously at itself. In distinguishing between *critical* reflection and other ways of reflecting, we recognize that reflection is a natural human activity. We all reflect and we do it often: many of us reflect silently to ourselves while walking home from work; we reflect at home with our families when we tell them about our day; we reflect in the car and in the bath; we even reflect in our dreams. Some of us write down our reflections in diaries or in on-line 'blogs'. Socrates is reported to have said that the unexamined life is not worth living. We would argue that the unexamined life is simply not feasible, and that unexamined practice can be both dangerous and unprofessional.

However, this book is not concerned merely with the day-to-day reflection that seems to be an intrinsic part of human experience. Indeed, such unstructured and unfocussed musings are not likely to produce anything recognized or valued by practitioners as evidence on which to base practice. Rather, our purpose in writing this book is to explore what we refer to as *critical* reflection. In choosing to use the word 'critical', we were mindful that it has certain negative connotations. The Oxford English Dictionary defines critical as 'expressing adverse or disapproving comments or judgments', and we certainly do not wish to give the impression that critical reflection should be either adverse or disapproving, despite the commonly held view that we should only reflect on aspects of our practice where things have gone wrong or which resulted in negative outcomes. This, for us, is absolutely not the case. Clearly, while it is possible to learn from our mistakes, there is also much to be gained from exploring positive aspects of our practice, and just as important, from examining the commonplace, everyday things that we usually do without giving them any thought at all.

The second dictionary definition of the term 'critical' is 'expressing or involving an analysis of the merits and faults of a literary or artistic work', and this is much closer to our intended meaning. Critical reflection goes beyond the simple recollection and description of events that usually characterize our everyday reflections, and involves some kind of analysis of the meanings and implications of what we are reflecting on. Now of course we are not suggesting that we never analyze situations and events when we reflect on our journey home from work or when we discuss our day with our family and friends. It is only human nature to try to find meaning in what we and others do and say. However, if we look again at the description that we cited above, we can see that, for us, critical reflection is both systematic and rigorous.

While reflection might not always be associated with rigour, there is a very good reason why we advocate a systematic approach in this book. As we have already observed, in the years since we wrote the first edition of this book, Evidence-Based Practice (EBP) has emerged as the dominant paradigm for the healthcare professions. EBP originated in medicine, and was devised as a way of replacing the opinions and beliefs of 'experts' with hard evidence from research (Evidence-Based Medicine Working Group, 1992). There has been a great deal of dispute and discussion in the intervening years about the role and status of so-called 'expert opinion' in making evidence-based decisions by practitioners about their own practice. While some writers, notably David Sackett, have argued that expert opinion can, in some cases, override the research evidence (Sackett et al., 1996), few writers regard the opinions of practitioners as a source of evidence in its own right, and those that do usually place it at the very bottom of the 'hierarchy of evidence' on which practice decisions are to be made. The view taken in this book is that many of the opinions of practitioners are grounded firmly in years of practical experience, and that these opinions can be a powerful source of evidence for informing their practice decisions. However, experience alone is rarely enough, and is not usually recognized by the EBP community as robust 'evidence' on which to base practice. One of the most important aims of this book is therefore to present critical reflection as a collection of methodologies and methods similar to existing and established research methodologies and methods for generating data, constructing knowledge and applying it to practice. In the case of critical reflection, our primary source of data is our own experiences, and data are generated and collated through the rigorous application of one or more systematic reflective frameworks, which constitute our data collection methods. As we shall see in subsequent chapters, these frameworks provide ways not only of collecting data through reflection on our experiences, but also incorporate methods of analyzing that data in order to generate knowledge and theory about practice. In short, we are suggesting that critical reflection is a way for practitioners to add to their evidence-base by conducting research into their own practice, and we are also offering ways in which they might begin to do this.

There are other reasons why we emphasize systems and rigour. Analysis is generally considered to be a high-level intellectual skill, and *self*-analysis of the kind demanded by critical reflection is doubly difficult. As many writers have pointed out, while we might have good intentions when examining our own thoughts, feelings and actions, it is normal and natural to subconsciously or unconsciously protect ourselves from some of the more personally uncomfortable conclusions that we might arrive at. Adhering rigorously to a systematic framework for reflection can prevent us (albeit subconsciously) from being selective in the aspects of a situation that we choose to examine. This is true not only for the negative elements of our practice. Some of us are quite ruthless with ourselves when it comes to identifying our own faults, but have difficulty in acknowledging our finer points. The use of a framework for reflection at least gives us a fighting chance of producing a well-rounded reflective analysis of a situation and of our role in shaping its outcome.

Other definitions of what counts as critical reflection share this concern with self-analysis and self-awareness. For example, the Frankfurt School of critical theory, led by Jürgen Habermas, sought to establish a new 'critical science' to stand alongside the empirical and hermeneutic sciences (Habermas, 1987). For Habermas, these three approaches to science are each driven by a 'cognitive interest' or basic human need to know, understand and act on the world. The empirical analytic sciences are the response to our 'technical' interest in the prediction and control of nature, the hermeneutic sciences are the response to our 'practical' interest in understanding one another, and the critical sciences are the response to our 'emancipatory' interest in freedom, including freedom both from outside social and political forces as well as from our own inner unconscious compulsions. For Habermas, to be critical is to be aware of, and alert to, the external and internal constraints and forces that prevent us from seeing the world as it really is. In the terminology of the critical theorists, this entails recognizing and challenging 'false consciousness', which can be overcome through perspective transformation, defined as:

> The emancipatory process of becoming critically aware of how and why the structure of psycho-cultural assumptions has come to constrain the way we see ourselves and our relationships, reconstituting this structure to permit a more inclusive and discriminating integration of experience and acting upon these new understandings (Mezirow, 1981, p. 6).

Habermas suggested that perspective transformation occurs through critical reflection, that is, the attempt to reveal the extent to which self-deception and ideology distort our perceptions.

Reflective moment

Think about a difficult or painful issue from your own practice which is now resolved. Try to recall your reflections about it at the time. In retrospect, now that you can be less emotional and more objective about the incident, can you think of any aspects of the issue that you avoided reflecting on at the time? Why do you think you might have avoided thinking about these aspects?

We discuss these ideas in more detail in Chapter 3, where we present them as one of several models of reflection. However, our concern in this book is not solely with reflection but with reflective practice, we are therefore also interested in models and frameworks that take us beyond self-awareness and the generation of theoretical evidence, and which provide opportunities for knowledge and theory to be applied back in a reflexive loop to the practice situation from which they originated. It is the frameworks within this *reflexive* model to which we pay particular attention, and this is the point at which, for us, theory and practice blend into the single act of reflexive practice. Once we reach this point, critical reflection is more than just another research methodology and becomes a paradigm for practice in its own right: a way of doing research-based practice in which the research and the practice occur simultaneously and represent the two sides of the same coin. Thus, critical reflection is for us not merely a means to the end of producing evidence. Our description of critical reflection in the first edition of our book talked about the reflective *process*, and we would wish to emphasize the benefits to be gained simply from *doing* reflection. Indeed, reflection is sometimes conducted verbally, and in these cases there is no tangible outcome, no written 'evidence' that the practitioner can refer back to. Even when reflections are written down, the writing is often a means to an end, a way of thinking more clearly where the value lies in the process of writing rather than what is actually written. Unlike most traditional forms of research, the process of doing critical reflection is often just as important as the outcomes it produces.

Conclusion

Many of the early definitions of reflection focused on its educational origins, and viewed it primarily as the attempt to learn from practice through 'retrospective contemplation' (see, for example, Palmer, Burns and Bulman, 1994). Other writers, most notably Johns, have taken Habermas' critical theory as their starting point and present reflection primarily as a means to self-knowledge and self-development. In fact, we are rapidly reaching the point at which reflection has become all things to all people, a catch-all term which encompasses everything from simple descriptions of their practice by beginning students, right through to Chris Johns' claim for the essence of reflection as simply 'a conscious decision to become' (Johns, 2006).

Our notion of *critical* reflection takes a somewhat different and rather more pragmatic approach. We began with the dictionary definition of the term 'critical' as being concerned with analysis, and we therefore presented critical reflection a means by which practitioners in the health and social care disciplines can analyze their experiences in order to generate evidence from their own practice, which can then be used to inform that practice. We also suggested that critical reflection can be regarded not only as a form of research, as a way for practitioners to conduct a critical inquiry into their own practice, but also as a reflexive integration of research and practice into a single act. In the following chapter we discuss and explore reflection as a practice paradigm to stand alongside evidence-based practice.

We might add that we regard critical reflection as an imperative; as an approach to practice that we feel can and should be adopted by all professional practitioners in health care. There is, perhaps, a potential conflict here: on the one hand we are presenting critical reflection as a high level intellectual activity involving the analysis, synthesis and evaluation of theory and knowledge, while on the other hand we are suggesting that critical reflection should become a part of the normal, everyday activity of all health care practitioners. However, we see no contradiction. In answer to our critics who claim that reflection is an advanced skill that can only be undertaken by practitioners with postgraduate degrees (see, for example, Wellard and Bethune, 1996; Teekman, 2000; Glaze, 2002), we would argue that there is no such thing as advanced practitioners, only *advancing* practitioners, and that critical reflection is simply one of many tools or methods which can help us all to advance further. Critical reflection is a difficult and challenging undertaking, but that is no reason for not attempting it.

The Oxford English Dictionary offers yet another definition of critical as 'having a decisive importance in the success or failure of something; crucial'. Critical reflection is therefore of *crucial* importance to our development as advancing practitioners. However, 'crucial' has a second meaning derived from its roots in the Latin word *crux*, meaning shaped like a cross. Critical reflection helps us with our *crucial* decisions, those decisions that we face every day when we stand at a crossroads and must decide between a number of different paths. Regardless of their magnitude and importance, choices present themselves to us constantly, and critical reflection offers a method for helping us to think and act in a mindful, considered and systematic way in order to make the crucial decisions that practice demands. In order to keep apace with the demands of practice, we must all become critical.

Reflective moment

Now turn back to the aims which you identified at the start of the chapter. To what extent have they been met? Write a paragraph outlining the knowledge you have acquired through reading this chapter and doing the exercises. Write a second paragraph identifying any aims which you feel were only partially met or not met at all. Divide your page into three columns. Head the first column 'What I need to learn', and make a list of any outstanding issues which you would like to learn more about. For example, you might wish to find out more about the Frankfurt School of critical science. Head the second column 'How I will learn it', and write down the ways in which your learning needs could be addressed; for example, through further reading, through attending study days, or through talking to other people. Head the third column 'How I will know that I have learnt it', and try to identify how you will know when you have met your needs.

You have just written your first learning plan for this book. We will be asking you to write one at the end of each chapter.

2

Knowledge and practice

Gary Rolfe

Introduction

We suggested in the previous chapter that critical reflection can be seen as a way of doing research, a way of doing practice or, preferably, as an amalgam of the two. This book can therefore be read as a handbook for doing practice, for doing research or for doing *praxis*, a form of research which is 'carried out by practitioners, improving practice by transforming the practice situation' (Rolfe, 1994).

This chapter begins by locating reflection firmly in the world of practice. Reflection that is not translated back into practice is of little use and is ultimately nothing more than an empty intellectual exercise. Reflection is presented as a paradigm for practice in the same vein as evidence-based practice, and is therefore concerned with making judgements about what counts as practice knowledge, how different forms of knowledge are to be valued and classified, and which research methods are best suited to generating that knowledge. The majority of this chapter is taken up with a philosophical discussion about different types of knowledge, the relationship between knowledge and practice, where knowledge comes from and how we might be confident about its accuracy and usefulness. It is, in other words, a gentle introduction to *epistemology*, the philosophical study of knowledge. Our aims for this chapter are:

1. to examine the claim that reflection is a paradigm for practice;
2. to explore and discuss different kinds of knowledge and think about their relationship to practice;

3. to think about where knowledge comes from and how it is generated; and
4. to begin to think more critically about yourself and your practice.

You might be tempted to skip this chapter, and it is possible to do so if you so wish. However, we have read too many books about reflection that start from the assumption that reflection is a good thing without properly examining why or without attempting to locate reflection within a wider remit of other paradigms and discourses. If you are happy to get to grips with the 'whats' and 'hows' of reflective practice without first considering the 'whys', then you can safely move on to Chapter 3. If, however, you wish to be able to argue the case for critical reflection as having a legitimate place alongside other discourses such as evidence-based practice (indeed, even if you only wish to understand what we mean by terms such as 'discourse'), then take a deep breath and jump in the deep end of this book.

Reflective moment

Think carefully about our aims for Chapter 2. Now think about your own practice and how these aims might contribute towards developing it.

Based on our aims above, identify write down some of your own aims, both in terms of what you hope to know and what you hope to be able to do after reading Chapter 2. We will return to these at the end of the chapter.

Reflective knowledge

Reflection is a process of thinking, feeling, imagining, and learning by considering what has happened in the past, what might have happened if things had been done differently, what is currently happening, and what could possibly happen in the future. Reflection might in some cases be a dispassionate and objective review of the facts of the matter, or it might focus predominantly on the feelings and personal reactions of the person who is reflecting or of someone else involved in the situation. While it is possible to reflect on what we or others did, might have done or failed to do, that is, on our actions and those of others, reflection is nevertheless a purely mental activity. And although there are various models, frameworks and techniques for teaching and enabling reflection, it is, in itself, of relatively little consequence for health and social care practitioners unless it is translated into positive outcomes in the real world. For that reason, this book is concerned not only with reflection, but with reflective and reflexive *practice*.

Whereas reflection is by definition a mental process, reflective practice, like evidence-based practice or advanced practice, is concerned with doing. As with evidence-based practice, it is a form of practice that is defined by its relationship to knowledge. Indeed, it might make more sense to consider evidence-based practice and reflective practice as *paradigms*, which Powers and Knapp (2006) define as organizing frameworks that contain:

- Concepts, theories, assumptions, beliefs, values, and principles that form a way for a discipline to interpret the subject matter with which it is concerned;
- Research methods considered to be best suited to generating knowledge within this frame of reference;
- What is open to investigation – priorities and views on knowledge deficit areas where research and theory building is most needed; and
- What is closed to enquiry for a time.

If we think of reflective practice as a paradigm, we can see that it is therefore not *only* concerned with doing. Reflective practice offers a complete framework for building knowledge and theory, including a view on what counts as knowledge, how it is generated and how it is to be disseminated. In other words, it is concerned with the nature of the relationship between thinking and doing.

Donald Schön (1983) compared the reflective paradigm with the traditional scientific paradigm of technical rationality, which he referred to as 'the Positivist epistemology of practice'. The most significant difference between reflective practice and technical rationality lies in the relationship between knowledge and practice. According to the epistemology of technical rationality, this relationship is predominantly one-way: knowledge is derived from decontextualized and objective scientific research and then applied to practice. This approach has in the past been referred to as research-based practice, and latterly as evidence-based practice (EBP), which is seen by many writers as the most recent manifestation of technical rationality. In contrast, the paradigm of reflective practice suggests a circular relationship in which the most important knowledge derives from practice itself through the process of reflection, and is then applied back to the situation from which it originated (Figure 2.1).

Figure 2.1 The paradigms of technical rationality and reflective practice

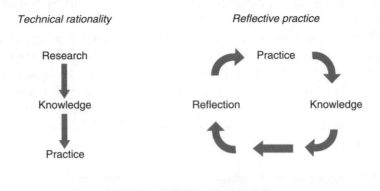

Reflective moment

Think about the similarities and differences between the two paradigms. What can you say about the relative importance of knowledge and theory in each? What are the implications of replacing research with reflection in the paradigm of reflective practice? Is it possible to practice safely and effectively without a research base?

We shall return to the relationship between knowledge and practice later in the chapter.

Disciplines, paradigms and discourses

We have seen that a discipline such as nursing or social work can accommodate a number of different paradigms (although one of these is usually dominant), and that these paradigms are more than simply frameworks for organizing knowledge. They also communicate judgements about what types of knowledge are considered 'best' or most useful, the most appropriate (or 'gold standard') methods for generating and disseminating that knowledge, and (often) the qualifications and accreditations required of the people who are authorized to do so. In many ways, the dominant paradigm can be seen as a collection of rules or laws by which members of a particular academic or practice discipline are expected to abide, and is therefore *disciplinary* in both meanings of the word. This imposition of discipline can be seen, for example, in the so-called 'hierarchies of evidence' of the technical rationality paradigm, which instructs academics on what methodologies to employ in their research studies, and practitioners on which types of knowledge (or evidence) they should apply to their practice.

Figure 2.2 Disciplines, paradigms and discourses

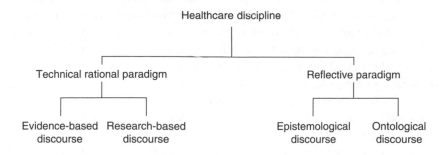

A *discipline* may host a several *paradigms*, and each paradigm may contain any number of *discourses* (Figure 2.2). The French writer and philosopher Michel Foucault, who had a particular interest in the ways that power and politics shape knowledge, described a discourse as the sum total of all the actual and possible conversations that could take place, or statements that could be made, concerning a particular subject (Foucault, 1980). The various discourses of reflective practice therefore include everything that can be meaningfully communicated about reflection within the confines of each particular discourse. We can see, then, that a discourse of reflective practice is created by our discussions and statements about reflective practice, but also that our discussions are determined by what has already been said, that is, by the discourse itself. For example, this book is adding to one or more discourses of reflective practice, but is also part of, and constrained by, the very discourses to which it is contributing. Foucault therefore proposed a circular or symbiotic relationship between the discourse and the subject of that discourse, where each feeds off the other. There is thus an intimate relationship between knowledge (the 'content' of a discourse or discipline) and power (the rules and procedures that determine how and by whom knowledge is defined, generated and disseminated within that discourse or discipline).

Theory and practice

In disciplines that include a practice component, discourses also need to take into account the conversations between theorists and practitioners. Some discourses, including many of those that are situated within the technical rationality paradigm, are somewhat one-sided in this respect. We saw earlier that the paradigm of technical rationality establishes a more or less one-way hierarchical relationship between research and practice and, by implication, between researchers and practitioners. Technical rationality discourses are therefore predominantly monologues rather than dialogues. In contrast, the reflective practice paradigm promotes the view that practitioners are also researchers into their own practice, and that knowledge from reflecting on practice has at least an equal status with knowledge from empirical scientific research. Thus, the circular and reflexive nature of reflective practice discourses suggests a rather different way of looking at the relationship between theorists and practitioners; as a true conversation between them rather than as a set of instructions passed from one to the other.

We can identify at least two distinct and separate discourses of reflective practice (see Figure 2.2), which Rolfe and Gardner (2006) have referred to as the epistemological (learning about our practice) and the ontological (learning about our self). These two discourses are epitomized by the following definitions or descriptions:

> [Reflection is] reviewing experience from practice so that it may be described, analysed, evaluated and consequently used to inform and change future practice. (Bulman and Schutz, 2008, p. 2)

> Reflection is not primarily a technology to produce better patient outcomes. Reflection is essentially about personal growth. (Johns, 2004, p. 44)

The epistemological discourse is concerned with reflection as a way of generating knowledge from and about practice which is used to bring about change in the situation from which it was generated. In contrast, the ontological discourse regards reflection as primarily concerned with exploring who we *are* as people and practitioners rather than with what we *know* about practice. That is not to say that it has no concern whatsoever with improving practice, but rather that, as Johns pointed out above, producing better patient outcomes is not its primary aim. Of course, there are other discourses which attempt to combine or integrate these positions, and yet others which fail to make a distinction between them.

While reflection as an exploration of self with a view to personal growth is a laudable aim, our concern in this book is primarily with the epistemological discourse: with reflection as a way of making sense of what we *do* rather than with who we *are*; with the production of knowledge from and for practice. However, we hope that we have demonstrated that there is no such thing as 'pure' or objective knowledge; that knowledge cannot stand apart from the 'political' system which authorizes and validates it. Thus, what is considered to be 'gold standard' knowledge in one paradigm might be completely disregarded by another. As Foucault maintained, knowledge and power cannot easily be separated; they are part and parcel of the same phenomenon, which he referred to as *power-knowledge* (Foucault, 1980).

Reflexive moment

We are all aware of Francis Bacon's dictum that knowledge is power, but Foucault suggests that the converse is also true – that power is knowledge. Think of some of the positions of power in your own discipline (university professors, journal editors, clinical managers, research grant funding bodies, etc.), and consider how they might influence what counts as knowledge, the relative importance of different types of knowledge, how knowledge is generated and disseminated, and so on. Think about how their power might be affected if our criteria for generating and judging knowledge were to change.

Thus, although this chapter is ostensibly an exploration of the relationship between knowledge and practice, it is also concerned very much with power relationships. For example, when we argue later in the chapter that practitioners should value and use knowledge from their own practice that they themselves have generated, we are also making a political statement about practitioners and power.

What is knowledge?

If, as we are claiming, one of the functions of reflection is to uncover or create knowledge from and about practice, then in order to understand fully the nature of reflection we must first explore what is meant and understood by the term 'knowledge'. Philosophers refer to the study of knowledge as *epistemology*, which can be defined simply as 'the philosophical theory of knowledge, which seeks to define it, distinguish its principal varieties, identify its sources, and establish its limits' (Bullock et al., 1988). Of these four tasks that epistemology has set itself, the first one of seeking to define knowledge is by far the most complicated, and is probably best left until last. Let us begin, then, with a look at the principal varieties of knowledge.

The principal varieties of knowledge

If you think about the ways that you use the word in everyday speech, it will quickly become apparent that 'knowledge' has a wide variety of uses and meanings. Philosophers often group these meanings into three types (Cardinal et al., 2004):

1. *Factual knowledge*, or what the philosopher Gilbert Ryle (1963) called *knowing that*. For example, knowing that bereaved people often pass through a series of stages of grieving is an example of factual knowledge. Factual knowledge plays an important part in theory construction and testing, and is therefore highly regarded in nursing and the helping professions. One of the important features of factual knowledge is that it can be expressed through language in the form of propositions or statements. For this reason, factual *knowing that* is often referred to as propositional knowledge.
2. *Practical knowledge*, or what Ryle (1963) referred to as *knowing how*. For example, knowing how to counsel a bereaved person is an example of practical knowledge. The practical knowledge of knowing how to do things is clearly very important in the caring professions, and has been studied by many theorists in these disciplines. Unlike factual knowledge, it is not always necessary to express practical knowledge through language. Indeed, philosophers such as Polanyi (1962) maintain that some practical knowledge, such as knowing how to ride a bicycle, is *tacit*, that is, unable to be expressed in words.
3. *Knowledge by acquaintance*, that is, knowing someone or something through direct contact with them, or what we might call *knowing who*. For example, knowing who Mr Jones is as a person is important if we are to offer him individualized counselling. Many health and social care practitioners regard knowledge by acquaintance as an extremely important prerequisite for their work, and therefore emphasize the importance of building therapeutic relationships as a way of coming to know and understand their clients and their individual needs.

There are other ways of categorizing the many different types of knowledge, but one of the interesting features of the above approach is that the three types are all exclusive of one another. So, for example, we might have factual knowledge about counselling (that is, we might know some theories about it, or we might have read in a book some facts about how to counsel a client) without having any practical knowledge whatsoever (we might never have actually counselled a client).

Alternatively, we might have a great deal of practical knowledge (we might have been involved in counselling many clients in the past) without having read a single book or journal paper. Similarly, we might be able to help a person with their grief simply by knowing them very well (they might be a friend, or we might have developed a good therapeutic relationship with them) without any knowledge or experience of counselling.

As a bereaved person, it is possible that I might encounter professional and lay helpers with a variety of combinations and permutations of these different types of knowledge. A friend or relative might be able to help me through my grief simply by knowing me as a person and therefore being aware of the kind of support that I most need at the time. An experienced but untrained health care worker might know the right things to say and do simply by having said and done them so many times before. And a student practitioner on her first practical placement might be able to help me by applying some of the counselling principles she has learnt in her lectures (such as being non-judgemental or adopting an 'open' posture) without having had any previous experience of working with bereaved people.

Clearly, though, people with a combination of all three types of knowledge will be of greatest help to me. We shall see, however, that although most writers would agree that all three types of knowledge are of use to practitioners in the health and social care professions, there are differences of opinion with regard to their relative importance, and once again, the politics of power plays an important role in determining the knowledge base of practice.

Reflective moment

Think of an example from your own practice of an interaction with a client. Try to identify all the different pieces of knowledge that you brought to the situation and categorize them according to whether they were 'knowing that', 'knowing how' or 'knowing who'. Which category did you draw on most and which did you draw on least? What does this tell you about your practice?

The sources of knowledge

The next issue of concern for epistemology is the question of where knowledge comes from. On the one hand, we can divide knowledge into that which arises from our experience (*a posteriori*) and that which was already present prior to experience (*a priori*). For example, we know that most clovers have three leaves *a posteriori* from our past experiences of seeing clovers and by hearing about other people's experiences of clovers. This notion that knowledge is derived and verified through observation and the senses is often referred to as *empiricism*. In contrast, our knowledge that triangles have three sides appears to have nothing to do with experience. Certainly, we do not have to go around counting the sides on actual triangles in order to verify this knowledge: it would appear to exist as a universal *a priori* truth independent of experience, something that can be worked out without reference to the senses. This notion that some knowledge can be arrived at through reasoning rather than observation is often referred to as *rationalism*. Applied to health care, we might consider the knowledge that many people grieve following bereavement as *a posteriori* or empirical, since it originates from our experiences. In contrast, the knowledge that grief is an unpleasant or painful emotion might be said to be *a priori* or rational, since it is part of the very essence of grief, and we do not have to experience grief to know that it causes us pain.

Although these two types of knowledge would appear to sit comfortably side by side, many empiricists would argue that we are born as *tabula rasa* or 'blank slates' and that *all* knowledge has its origin in our subsequent experiences of the outside world; in other words, all knowledge is empirical. Empiricism accounts for the apparently *a priori* knowledge of mathematics and geometry by arguing that such knowledge is not innate, but is learnt implicitly as we learn language. Thus, while it might appear that the fact that triangles have three sides is known to us prior to any experience with actual triangles, the empiricists would argue that it is a fact *by definition*, and that we have learnt the definition of a triangle through our experience of learning language. The empiricists would therefore dispute the claim that we already know that grief causes us pain prior to our experience. They would claim that although we do not have to experience grief to understand the pain it causes, the knowledge that grief causes pain is learnt when we learn what the word grief means. We are therefore not born with this knowledge; it is acquired with our knowledge of language and the meaning of words.

This assertion that all knowledge comes to us through our senses suggests that we must look outward rather than inside ourselves to learn about the world, and is the starting point for the empirical sciences. Of course, many reflective practitioners also start with experience, although it tends to be prior experience, and they attempt to gain access to it by looking inwards rather than outwards. Some reflective practitioners might be described more as rationalists than empiricists, since they believe that at least some of their practice knowledge is innate and prior to experience; perhaps emanating from an essential 'inner self', from an internal *a priori* moral consciousness, or perhaps resulting from spiritual or quasi-religious inner experiences. Yet others object to the term 'rationalist' to describe this source of seemingly intuitive inner knowledge, preferring to regard themselves as non- or even anti-rationalists. Conversely, some scientists maintain that there is a role for *a priori* knowledge as part of the scientific method, arguing for example that whereas hypothesis testing relies on empiricism, the generation of hypotheses is sometimes non-empirical and based in rationalism or intuition.

We can see, then, that the reflective paradigm (and particularly the epistemological discourse of reflection) shares a number of similarities with scientific empiricism. However, although both concur that practitioners' knowledge derives mainly (or even entirely) from experience, there are clear differences concerning the most important types, with the scientific paradigm privileging factual 'knowing that' and the reflective paradigm favouring practical 'knowing how' and personal 'knowing who'.

Reflective moment

Using the same example from your own practice, try to identify where your knowledge came from. How much of it was rational or *a priori* and how much was empirical? What does this tell you about your practice?

The limits of knowledge

If we accept that most of what we know comes to us through our senses, then it is tempting to think that we can be fairly certain of our knowledge; that 'seeing is believing'. However, philosophers have identified a number of reasons for being cautious about what it is possible to know in this way. Even if we accept for the moment that our senses are to be trusted and that seeing actually *is* believing, knowledge of what is currently before our eyes is of limited practical use to us. As practitioners, we need to be able to generalize and predict; that is, to

Figure 2.3 Generating knowledge through induction and deduction

many individual **induction** → general law **deduction** → specific case
observations

Every clover I have seen   *All clovers have*   *The next clover I*
has three leaves   *three leaves*   *see will have three*
leaves

use the knowledge presented to us in the here-and now to attempt to understand the there-and-then; to use the knowledge gleaned from *this* situation with *this* client to know about future encounters with similar clients, and indeed, to be able to say something about *all* encounters with *all* clients. In fact, successful health and social care practice depends on the ability to reason from particular instances to general rules or laws (what philosophers refer to as induction), and then to use those general laws in order to make predictions about future particular instances (deduction).

We can demonstrate this process by returning to an earlier example (Figure 2.3). Every one of the many clovers that I have ever seen growing in my garden, in public parks and elsewhere has had three leaves. From this empirical knowledge I can *induce* the general law that all clovers have three leaves, and from this general inductive law I can then *deduce* or predict that any clover I come across in the future will also have three leaves. Of course, the flaws in this logic are immediately apparent: just because I have never experienced a clover with four leaves does not preclude its existence. The philosopher David Hume identified this *problem of induction* in the eighteenth century, noting that the past can never be a certain predictor of the future. In the twentieth century, Karl Popper extended the argument to show that even modern *scientific* knowledge based on the logic of induction can never be certain, and that there is thus no such thing as a scientific 'law'. In other words, even though a new drug has been tested on thousands of subjects in the most rigorous of clinical trials and found to be safe, there is no guarantee that it will be safe for everyone. And even if it was tested on the entire population of the world, there are new people being born all the time.

Even if we do assume that our inductive general knowledge provides us with more or less accurate information about how people in general behave and react, this knowledge is of little use to us as practitioners unless we are able to make deductions from it right down to the individual level; that is, we need to be sure that the general knowledge applies to our specific practice with the individual client in front of us at that moment. However, just as there is a problem with induction from the specific to the general, so too is there a problem with deduction from the general back to the individual. The problem is that general inductive knowledge is usually decontextualized: in order for it to apply to all cases in all situations, the influence of the specific individuals and locations involved in its generation have to be nullified or cancelled out. But that in turn relies on the assumption that all people in all situations will respond in a uniform manner to the same intervention. Where drugs are concerned, that might well be the case: we can reasonably assume that everyone will respond in more or less the same way to the same drug, regardless of who administers it, where it is administered, and so on (although even here we need to take into account the 'placebo effect'). However, it is perhaps not possible to make the same assumption when it comes to non-physical interventions of the type that many health and social care practitioners perform on a daily basis. For example, to what extent does our general knowledge of how bereaved people respond to a particular form of counselling apply to how a particular client will respond on a particular day in a particular setting to a particular counsellor?

Even if we accept the inductive logic of using our empirical knowledge of individual cases in order to arrive at general knowledge about all cases and the deductive logic of using these laws to make specific predictions about new individual cases, we are still working on the assumption that this empirical knowledge is accurate in the first place. A major problem for philosophers with the idea of empirical knowledge is how we can be sure that any knowledge gained through the senses is true or accurate. On the one hand, few people would deny that, at least some of the time, our senses can deceive us. For example, most of us have been fooled by optical illusions and even by hallucinations. This realization that we can *sometimes* be fooled led the French philosopher René Descartes to ponder on the possibility that we might *always* be fooled (perhaps by some powerful supernatural being), that the world might not be as it seems (my perceptions might be permanently distorted), or indeed that it might not exist at all (I might be dreaming). As well as the question of whether what we see and hear is accurate (reliability), there is also the issue of whether it is true (validity). For example, when Mr Jones tells me that he is feeling upset, I might be relatively certain that I heard him correctly or that I was not suffering from an auditory hallucination, but I still cannot be certain that he really is upset since, for a variety of possible reasons, he might not be telling me the truth. This is equally problematic whether Mr Jones is telling me about his distress in response to a general enquiry about his state of mind, in response to a question during a qualitative research interview, or by ticking a box on a Likert scale questionnaire.

Further reading

Daniel Cardinal and colleagues (2004) have published a very readable introduction to epistemology that is an ideal starting point for further detail on all of the issues discussed in this chapter. Similar ground is covered by Peter Cole (2002) in his book *The Theory of Knowledge*. For a more in-depth understanding of empiricism, you might wish to look at Meyers' book (2006), particularly the introduction where he contrasts empiricism with rationalism, and Chapter 5 on empiricism and the *a priori*. Inductive and deductive reasoning and their relation to evidence for practice are discussed in Phelan and Reynolds' book (1996) *Argument and Evidence*, particularly in Chapter 12, and by Garnham and Oakhill (1994) in Chapters 5 and 7.

The scientific community has attempted to address these problems by setting strict limits firstly on how knowledge can be produced, and secondly on who is qualified and entitled to produce and disseminate it. In the first case, the reliability and validity of knowledge is safe-guarded by the researcher having to adhere to the rigours of methodology, whether it be the strict controls governing a randomized controlled trial or the self-auditing processes of a phenomenological study. In this way, the risk is minimized that the subjective experiences of the researcher might distort the data, and that the person supplying the data is being deceitful. In the second case, restrictions may be placed on who is allowed to access funding for large research studies, on who might be employed as a researcher, or even on who might be permitted to teach and disseminate research findings. Generally speaking, a doctoral degree would be required as proof that the individual had undertaken the appropriate research training, or else the person would need to be overseen by a suitably qualified supervisor. We can see, then, how knowledge and power interact, and how the technical rationality paradigm attempts to control and regulate knowledge production and dissemination.

In contrast, the paradigm of reflective practice places few limits and restrictions on the production and dissemination of knowledge. Although there are a number of frameworks for reflection, they are largely optional and do not provide the same safeguards against subjectivity and inaccuracy as the research methodologies which are approved by the scientific paradigm. For this reason, a number of criticisms have been levelled at the reflective practice paradigm by members of the scientific community, with claims that the knowledge obtained through reflection is inferior to that obtained by traditional research methods. First, it is argued that reflective practice is unsound because there is no generalizable research evidence to show its effectiveness (Carroll et al., 2002, Mackintosh, 1998). Secondly it is suggested that the knowledge obtained from reflection might be subject to unwitting bias and distortion due, for example, to problems of faulty or selective recall (Newell, 1992; Reece Jones, 1995). Third, it has been argued (Cox, 2002) that some reflective practitioners, particularly students, might deliberately distort or even make up the content of their reflections to further their own needs, perhaps in order to pass an assignment or to justify their actions.

Reflective moment

Think about some of the things that you have learnt about yourself and your practice through reflecting on it. How certain can you be of its accuracy or truthfulness? Do you trust the results of your reflections more or less than you trust the knowledge you obtain from research journals? Why?

There are clearly problems in judging one paradigm according to the standards of another, and Rolfe (2005c) has attempted to show how all of these objections to reflective practice can equally be applied to the paradigm of technical rationality itself. It must be remembered, though, that there are limitations to any method of knowledge production, whether it is the randomized controlled trial (RCT) or reflection on practice. In the former case, generalizability and objectivity are gained at the expense of local relevance and subjective interest. We have already seen that the large decontextualized RCT, conducted by the disinterested, objective researcher, is very useful for making general statements about populations, but can only be applied accurately to individual cases if the assumption is made that each case is essentially the same as every other. While this might indeed be true for the efficacy of a drug, many healthcare practitioners will argue that each therapeutic encounter with each of their patients or clients is unique and cannot be predicted in advance from the findings of RCTs.

We can see, then, that there is a place in the healthcare practitioner's repertoire for all three types of knowledge discussed above; that is, factual or propositional knowledge from scientific research, practical knowledge from reflecting on previous experiences, and knowledge by acquaintance from building therapeutic relationships with patients and clients. Each is produced in different ways, each has particular strengths and weaknesses, and each has a part to play in building up an overall picture from which to make clinical decisions. We might go further and argue that each is a type of evidence, and that evidence-based practice depends on all three if wise clinical judgements are to be made. It makes little sense, then, to suggest that certain types of knowledge are better than others, or that the various methods for producing knowledge should be arranged in a hierarchy with some having gold standard status and others being relegated to the bottom.

Definitions of knowledge

We can now begin to pull these threads together in order to arrive at some definitions of knowledge. We will begin by offering the traditional view that knowledge is *justified true belief*. Thus, for something to count as knowledge, it must first be believed by the person making the knowledge claim. It makes no sense to say, for example, that 'I know the world is round but I don't believe it'. To *know* something is, first and foremost, to believe it to be true. This criterion of belief has some interesting implications, since a belief is personal to whoever holds it. You and I might have completely different beliefs and, hence, different knowledge bases: I might 'know' that the world is round, whereas you 'know' that it is flat. So does that mean that it is possible for two people to know contradictory things about the same object? Surely at least one of us must be wrong.

This brings us to the second criterion for knowledge, which is the thorny issue of truth. Knowledge is not just any belief; it is *true* belief. The difficulty here is that there are many ways of defining what is to count as truth. On the one hand, there is the 'realist' view that truth implies a correspondence with some sort of external reality: that the statement 'the world is round' is true if, and only if, the world *really is round*. This might seem to be no more than common sense, but the problem is how such judgements about reality are to be made. Let us take a different example to illustrate this point. According to the realists, the statement 'democracy is a good thing' is true if and only if democracy really is a good thing. But how can we judge whether it really is? Surely, it could be argued, reality is all around us, and we only need to look and listen in order to see and hear the truth. As we have seen above, however, this supposes that our senses never lie to us, that we perceive the world directly and without distortion and that the subjects of our observations always tell the truth. Unfortunately, psychologists tell us otherwise: they are easily able to demonstrate, through a variety of optical, auditory and tactile illusions, ways in which our senses constantly fool us. We can never be certain that what we perceive through our senses is how the world really is, and many philosophers, psychologists and sociologists, as well as some physicists, believe that all of our perceptions are 'theory-laden', that we see the world according to how we expect to see it. The difficulty for the realist view of truth, then, is that if we have no objective and direct access to reality; then we have nothing against which to judge our truth claims.

This has led some thinkers to suggest an alternative view of truth, which we might loosely term anti-realist or *constructivist*, which argues that truth is created in the minds of people rather than discovered in the outside world. So, for example, the statement 'democracy is a good thing' is true because we have decided that it is true. The constructivists do not believe that 'the truth is out there', but rather that it is 'in here' in individual minds. That is not to say that each of us has a totally different conception of truth, but that we collectively decide as a society what is to count as true for us. It also means that truths are not eternal; they are not true for all time, but can shift along with our perceptions of the world. Seen in this way, truth takes on a political dimension, and the question we should ask ourselves is not 'is this true?' but rather 'who decides whether this is true?'

This brings us to our third criterion of knowledge, which is that our true belief must be supported by some form of evidence: to count as knowledge it must be a *justified* true belief. It is not enough to say 'I know the world is round, but I can't (or won't) tell you how I know it'. I must offer proof. For the realists, the justification of the truth of a statement takes the form of some kind of demonstration that the statement corresponds to objective reality. So, for example, I can demonstrate that the world is round by setting sail in a westerly direction and continuing in a straight line until I eventually return to the point that I started from. I can demonstrate that democracy is a good thing by conducting surveys of life in democratic and undemocratic countries and comparing the two. This approach to justification supposes that there is a method by which we can gain access to reality which can somehow overcome all the difficulties mentioned above; that there is an *objective* method which can avoid all the subjective pitfalls such as optical and auditory illusions and other distortions introduced by imperfect individual observers and reporters. Most realists argue that the best and most objective method for perceiving reality is the method of science. Some, who often call themselves *positivists* (after Comte 1988), argue that the method of science can be applied not only to the physical world, but also to the social world, and even to the study of individual people.

The constructivists, however, would argue that such an approach does not set the search for truth (and, hence, for knowledge) on an objective footing; all that it does is to shift the political decision as to what counts as truth back a stage. Rather than ask the question 'who decides what is to count as truth?', we must now ask 'who decides what is to count as the best method for determining what counts as truth?' The constructivists would therefore call into question the decision to accept science as the best or only way of gaining access to the truth, and would see it as a politically loaded decision taken and maintained by a small group of people who have a great deal to lose if the criteria for truth and knowledge were to change. As Foucault (1980) pointed out, if knowledge is constructed by people, then certain people have the power to define what counts as knowledge, who is qualified to undertake the task of generating knowledge, what count as acceptable ways of doing so, who is qualified to disseminate that knowledge, and in which ways. The constructivists therefore argue that scientific research has been chosen as the dominant method for generating knowledge not for any objective reason, but for reasons of power.

Further reading

As before, Cardinal et al. (2004) offer a clear and concise overview of definitions of knowledge. Books that deal simply and clearly with constructivism are hard to find, but the topic is explored and explained in some depth by Vivien Burr (1995) in her book An *Introduction to Social Constructionism*. Evans and Hardy (2010) have written a very useful book for social workers on how to apply different types of knowledge to practice and Thompson's (2000) book *Theory and Practice in Human Services* covers similar ground in a more generic way.

Knowledge and practice

One of the problems for any practice-based discipline with accepting scientific knowledge as the dominant form is that it implies a particular model of the relationship between knowledge and practice. As we saw earlier from Figure 2.1, this technical rationality paradigm supposes a simple hierarchy with knowledge and theory at the top, and practice at the bottom. In the terminology of Gilbert Ryle (1963), it suggests that 'knowing that' precedes and informs 'knowing how'; that we must first learn the theory before applying it to practice. This in turn suggests a parallel hierarchy with researchers and theorists at the top and practitioners at the bottom.

We have already suggested a number of limitations inherent in the paradigm of technical rationality. First, of course, we have argued that practice based solely or predominantly on propositional knowledge from the findings of empirical research is incomplete, since it downplays the vast repertoire of experiential knowledge that many writers (Benner, 1984; Dreyfus and Dreyfus, 1986) would see as the defining feature of expertise. Second, and as a direct consequence of this, it devalues the role of the practitioner to that of a technician whose job is merely to apply the knowledge of other people, many of whom have not practiced healthcare for some considerable time. Third, while factual 'knowing that' can contribute to theory-building, it does not have the same relationship to practice as practical 'knowing how'. It is one thing to know *that* a patient requires CPR, but quite another matter to know *how* to administer it. Fourth, most knowledge derived from empirical research is decontextualized and generalizable; that is, it is general knowledge which applies to populations rather than individuals, to people rather than persons. It takes account neither of the unique interpersonal relationships that comprise healthcare practice, nor of the unique and idiosyncratic settings in which that practice takes place.

The reflective paradigm offers an alternative approach to practice in which knowing and doing are closely linked, and in which the knowledge inherent in practice can be examined and explored by the practitioner by reflecting on past experiences and then applying them to future practice. In other words, the reflective paradigm values 'knowing how' as equal in importance to 'knowing that', and offers ways for the practitioner to uncover and articulate their own experiential knowledge as a valid source of evidence for practice. It also places emphasis on the unique clinical encounter between the individual practitioner and the individual patient. The reflective paradigm therefore offers a way for practitioners to take control of their own body of experiential knowledge and lays the foundations for a new individualized approach to evidence-based practice in which the evidence acquired through reflection has an equal status with evidence from large-scale empirical research. In the next chapter we will explore the reflective paradigm in more detail, looking particularly at the methods and methodologies it employs for generating knowledge from reflection.

Reflective moment

Now turn back to the aims which you identified at the start of the chapter. To what extent have they been met? Write a paragraph outlining the factual and practical knowledge you have acquired through reading this chapter and doing the exercises. Write a second paragraph identifying any aims which you feel were only partially met or not met at all. As in the previous chapter, divide your page into three columns. Head the first column 'What I need to learn', and make a list of any outstanding issues which you would like to learn more about. For example, you might wish to find out more about the inductive and deductive methods. Head the second column 'How I will learn it', and write down the ways in which your learning needs could be addressed; for example, through further reading, through attending study days, or through talking to other people. Head the third column 'How I will know that I have learnt it', and try to identify how you will know when you have met your needs.

3

Models and frameworks for critical reflection

Gary Rolfe

Introduction

We saw from Chapter 2 that the paradigm of reflective practice offers an alternative way of thinking and doing for nurses and healthcare practitioners which complements the technical rationality paradigm. Whereas technical rationality provides generalizable evidence for practice from empirical research, reflection enables practitioners to generate their own unique body of personal knowledge directly from their own practice. We also saw that there is a close relationship between knowledge and power, and so reflective practice also suggests the possibility of a shift in power and control over the health and social care disciplines from academic researchers to practitioners themselves. Put simply, the cognitive or epistemological discourse of reflective practice discussed in the previous chapter offers a way for the practitioner's own experiences to be taken seriously alongside research findings as a source of evidence on which to base practice.

It is, at least in part, this ability to generate knowledge from practice rather than relying on external research findings that establishes health and social care practitioners as professionals in their own right rather than as merely technologists who apply knowledge generated and disseminated by others. True professionals have a full and bilateral relationship with knowledge: they not only apply knowledge to their practice, but they also generate and disseminate it; that is, they are researchers and educationalists as well as practitioners. For some, this full professional role will be achieved through participation in formal research projects or by working part time as lecturers in an educational establishment. However, for the majority of practitioners, their research and educational roles are best achieved through reflecting on their own practice and by encouraging and facilitating colleagues and students to do the same through mentorship and clinical supervision.

In order for reflective practice to function as an alternative to the technical rationality paradigm, it must be seen as more than merely *ad hoc*; reflection and reflective practice requires some structure in the form of methodologies and methods. There are a number of reasons why a formal structure is necessary. The first reason is *political*: just as the technical rationality paradigm controls and regulates knowledge by accrediting certain research methodologies as valid and reliable, so must the reflective paradigm establish criteria that reflective methodologies must meet in order to produce valid and reliable reflective knowledge. Linked to this is the *professional* reason: as well as the internal regulation of knowledge production, the healthcare professions must also demonstrate to other professions, to prospective healthcare practitioners, to patients and clients, and to the outside world in general that there are mechanisms in place for generating valid and reliable knowledge for and from practice. In addition, there is the *practical* reason of providing structure and guidelines to the reflective process in order to facilitate practitioners to undertake it with skill and confidence, and also the *personal* reason of offering a range of methods and methodologies to suit the preferences of individual practitioners. Our aims for this chapter are:

1. to examine the political, professional, practical and personal drivers for a reflective paradigm;
2. to discuss and analyze three models for reflection;
3. to explore a number of reflective frameworks associated with each of the models; and
4. to examine in depth a number of reflexive frameworks based on Kolb's model of reflexive learning.

Reflective moment

Think carefully about our aims for Chapter 3. Now think about your own practice and how these aims might contribute towards developing it.

Based on our aims above, identify and write down some of your own, both in terms of what you hope to know and what you hope to be able to do after reading Chapter 3. We will return to these at the end of the chapter.

Models and frameworks of reflection

Whereas researchers refer to broad methodologies such as ethnography or surveys, and specific methods such as participant observation or postal questionnaires, reflective practitioners often talk about models and frameworks. When we refer in this chapter to *models*, we mean the broad philosophical theories and assumptions that underpin a particular approach to reflection. *Frameworks* are specific methods or approaches that provide help and guidance (perhaps in the form of cue questions or headings) for reflecting within a chosen model. In our experience, many writers and practitioners confuse models and frameworks, in the same way that many researchers confuse methodologies with methods. This can lead to the *ad hoc* use of inappropriate reflective frameworks for the task in hand and a mix-and-match approach that might not provide the most effective way to reflect on a particular situation. Just as it is important for the researcher to understand the principles, assumptions and appropriate data collection methods of their chosen methodology, so too should the reflective practitioner understand the principles, assumptions and appropriate reflective frameworks of their chosen model of reflection. In this chapter we will explore three models or philosophies (methodologies) of reflection along with some of the more common frameworks (methods) associated with each of them. In keeping with our focus on the epistemological discourse of reflection (see Figure 2.2), we will not be discussing 'ontological' models such as that advocated by Chris Johns, which regard the primary aim of reflection as personal growth or development.

Dewey's model of reflective learning

The most common philosophical position, around which many of the more familiar frameworks are constructed, is most clearly expressed by the American psychologist, educationalist and philosopher John Dewey

Figure 3.1 Dewey's model of reflective learning

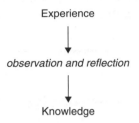

Experience

↓

observation and reflection

↓

Knowledge

Source: Dewey, J., *Experience and Education* (1938) reproduced with permission of Kappa Delta Pi, International Honor Society in Education.

in his claim that 'we learn by doing and realising what came of what we did' (Dewey, 1938). Dewey was an early advocate of learning by discovery and was critical of the so-called 'spectator theory of knowledge' which placed the knower at a distance and separate from the thing to be known. In contrast, Dewey regarded knowing as an active dialectical process in which knowledge resulted from a personal engagement with the world. Seen this way, knowledge is not a thing that we can possess: to have knowledge of something is to have the ability to engage with it through enquiry. Sometimes this enquiry is immediate and first-hand, as when a child learns to ride a bicycle by doing it, but at other times the enquiry is retrospective and comes about after the event. The basic assumption of this model is therefore that knowledge can be constructed through active reflection on current or past experiences; that experience can somehow be processed and converted into knowledge, much as the raw data from empirical research studies can be processed statistically or thematically into useful findings (Figure 3.1).

We can see the philosophy underpinning Dewey's model of learning in a number of definitions of reflective practice. For example, Fitzgerald (1994, p. 67) defines reflection as 'The retrospective contemplation of practice undertaken in order to uncover the knowledge used in a particular situation, by analysing and interpreting the information recalled'.

There have been a number of attempts to construct methods or frameworks of reflection based on Dewey's model, and one of the most commonly employed in healthcare practice is that offered by Gibbs (1988).

Gibbs asks us to pay attention to three particular aspects of the situation. First, we must describe what happened, and consider what we thought and how we felt at the time. Second, we must apply our critical faculties to the situation; we must evaluate the good and bad

Figure 3.2 Gibbs' reflective framework

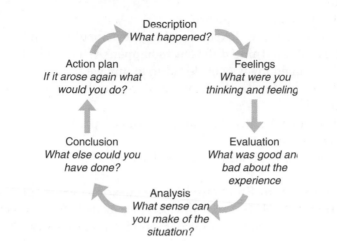

Description
What happened?

Feelings
*What were you
thinking and feeling*

Action plan
*If it arose again what
would you do?*

Evaluation
*What was good an
bad about the
experience*

Conclusion
*What else could you
have done?*

Analysis
*What sense can
you make of the
situation?*

Source: Gibbs (1988).

points and attempt to make sense of it. Third, we must consider what else we could have done at the time, and what we might do in the future if the situation arose again. You might notice that these cues are rather general and unspecific. This has the advantage of giving the framework a somewhat generic feel, although some (particularly novice) reflective practitioners might find it rather too vague. Furthermore, although it is set out as a cycle, the process would appear to terminate with the 'action plan', and it is not clear how this phase links back to the 'description'.

Sarah Stephenson (Holm and Stephenson 1994) offered a similar, if somewhat more detailed, framework. Stephenson developed this framework as part of her degree studies while working as a staff nurse at the John Radcliffe Hospital in Oxford. As she points out, 'Unlike writing an essay, there are no definitive rules on how to reflect. No one method is universally correct' (Holm and Stephenson 1994). She therefore went about constructing her own set of cue questions, primarily as a tool to structure her own reflective writing.

Choose a situation
Ask yourself:

- What was my role in this situation? Did I feel comfortable or uncomfortable? Why?
- What actions did I take? How did I and others act? Was it appropriate?

- How could I have improved the situation for myself, the patient, my mentor?
- What can I change in future?
- Do I feel as if I have learnt anything new about myself?
- Did I expect anything different to happen? What and why?
- Has it changed my way of thinking in any way?
- What knowledge from theory and research can I apply to this situation?
- What broader issues, for example ethical, political or social, arise from this situation?
- What do I think about these broader issues?

You will see that Stephenson's cue questions are somewhat more specific than Gibbs', and that initially the focus is far more on action than on conceptualization and theorizing. In many ways, this framework is more faithful to Dewey's imperative of learning by thinking about what came of our actions, since Stephenson begins by asking us to consider what we did and how we might do it differently, and only then moves on to ask us to examine our own practice knowledge along with the broader knowledge and theory base.

However, a limitation of both of these frameworks as ways of doing practice is their emphasis on thinking at the expense of doing. Knowledge arises out of reflection on past actions, but there are no guidelines or cue questions to help practitioners to apply that knowledge back to practice beyond asking them to think about what they would do if the situation arose again. However, as Atkins and Murphy point out, 'For reflection to make a real difference to practice, it is important that the outcome includes a commitment to action' (Atkins and Murphy, 1994, p. 51). Such a commitment appears to be absent in both of these frameworks. This is perhaps unsurprising since Gibbs is an educationalist and Stephenson's framework was developed primarily in the classroom as a structure for writing reflective assignments rather than in the practice arena. We might therefore describe the frameworks based on Dewey's model as concerned with the cognitive or educational aspect of reflection rather than directly with reflective practice.

Habermas' model of critical reflection

Jürgen Habermas, one of the most influential sociologists and philosophers of the second half of the twentieth century, applied the understandings of the Frankfurt School of critical theory to knowledge generation and reflection. Habermas (1974) argued that there are three primary areas in which human interest generates or constitutes knowledge, which he referred to as the technical, practical and emancipatory. The *technical* domain is concerned with the human interest in control and manipulation of the environment, and incorporates many of the technical and scientific disciplines and modes of thought. The *practical* domain is concerned with social interaction and the understanding of meaning, and broadly incorporates the humanities and social sciences. The *emancipatory* domain is concerned largely with what Habermas terms 'self-knowledge', that is, knowledge of the self in relation to social and institutional forces of control. The emancipatory domain is the field of study that aims to provide a transcendental perspective or subjective overview through the critical sciences, which include psychoanalysis, feminist theory and Marxist philosophy. The goal of the emancipatory domain is therefore self-emancipation from 'false consciousness' (that is, the point of view imposed by external social and psychological structures) through critical reflection, which leads to a 'perspective transformation' in which the world is seen as it really is.

The focus of critical reflection is therefore the transformation of the way that practitioners view the world and their place in it, and is summarized in the definition of reflection offered by Boyd and Fales (1983, p. 101) 'The process of creating and clarifying the meaning of experience in terms of self in relation to both self and the world. The outcome of this process is changed conceptual perspectives'.

Habermas' model of critical reflection has been extended and applied to nursing and midwifery by Beverley Taylor. Although Habermas associated reflection primarily with the emancipatory domain, Taylor's framework describes the activities associated with three types of reflection, corresponding to each of Habermas' three domains (Table 3.1), arguing that 'no type of reflection is better than another; each has its own value for different purposes' (Taylor, 2006, p. 103).

Table 3.1 Taylor's framework for critical reflection

	Technical reflection	*Practical reflection*	*Emancipatory reflection*
Reflective activities	Assessing and planning Implementing Evaluating	Experiencing Interpreting Learning	Constructing Deconstructing Confronting Reconstructing

Source: Adapted from Taylor (2006).

Taylor (2006, p. 139) further broke down each of these reflective activities into a series of questions. For example, the activity of 'experiencing' in the practical reflection domain included the following questions:

- What was happening?
- When was it happening?
- Where was it happening?
- Why was it happening?
- Who was involved?
- How were you involved?
- What was the setting like, in terms of its smells, sounds and sights?
- What were the outcomes of the situation?
- How did you feel honestly about the situation?

We can see, then, that Taylor's framework provides a very comprehensive and highly structured format for critical reflection.

Hesok Susie Kim (1999) has also produced a framework based on the work of Habermas for what she referred to as 'critical reflective inquiry'. Although Kim's framework was designed primarily to be employed by reflective researchers as a method of data collection, she pointed out that it is equally applicable to reflection on practice by the practitioners themselves (Table 3.2). Kim's framework is less prescriptive than Taylor's, and does not offer cue questions. However, she has provided some fairly detailed instructions for how it might be used in practical settings.

Table 3.2 Kim's framework for critical reflective inquiry

	Descriptive phase	Reflective phase	Critical/emancipatory phase
Processes	• Descriptions of practice events (actions, thoughts and feelings)	• Reflective analysis against espoused theories (scientific, ethical and aesthetic)	• Critique of practice regarding conflicts, distortions and inconsistencies
	• Examination of descriptions for genuineness and comprehensiveness	• Reflective analysis of situations • Reflective analysis of intentions	• Engagement in emancipatory and change process
Products	• Descriptive narratives	• Knowledge about practice processes and applications • Self-awareness	• Learning and change in practice • Self-critique and emancipation

Source: Kim, H.S. (1999) reproduced with permission of the *Journal of Advanced Nursing*.

Kim's framework echoes Habermas' areas of human interest, and breaks down reflection into three phases, starting with a descriptive phase in which:

> Descriptive narratives of specific instances of practice in specific clinical situations are written or constructed by nurses, including the descriptions of nurses' actions, thoughts and feelings, as well as the circumstances and features of the situations. (Kim, 1999, p. 1207)

The aim of these narratives is 'to open a door that has been closed behind, and to look back into the past' (Kim, 1999), and it is the job of the facilitator (or, in Kim's model, the researcher) first to keep the narratives at the descriptive level, and second to help the practitioner to 'identify what is missing in the descriptions to make them comprehensive and complete' (Kim, 1999).

In the second (reflective) phase, these descriptive narratives are 'examined in a reflective mode against practitioners' personal beliefs, assumptions and knowledge' (Kim, 1999). The aim here is for practitioners to uncover their 'espoused theories' relating to the specific situation, so that they 'can discover not only how [they are] able to handle complex situations but also in what ways [they] become entrenched in routinized practice' (Kim, 1999). In other words, the reflective phase of the process enables practitioners to begin to build their own personal and situational knowledge and theory base so that they are able to respond not only from their scientific knowledge, but also from their experiential knowledge.

However, Kim argued that it is not enough merely to construct knowledge from practice settings, and that the practitioner must also reflect on how that knowledge can lead to intentions to act; in other words, how experiential knowledge translates into clinical actions. She pointed out that this is extremely difficult for the practitioner to do alone, and usually requires facilitation, since 'it is not easy for people to free themselves from "rationalizations" they make of their actions and partition out which actions were intended from which actions were not intended' (Kim, 1999).

Kim's third and final 'critical/emancipatory' phase builds on the insights into practice acquired in the reflective phase and 'is oriented to correcting and changing less-than-good or ineffective practice, or moving forward to future assimilation of new innovations emerging from practice' (Kim, 1999). In this phase, the facilitator and the practitioner 'engage in the process of critique in order to point out problems that require change in practice' (Kim, 1999). The required changes can be either personal or communal, but ultimately require both self-knowledge and self-emancipation, since:

> Through the [facilitator's] questioning and probing, practitioners can engage in self-dialogue and argumentation with themselves in order to clarify validity claims embedded in their actions, bringing forth the hidden meanings and disguises that systematically result in self-oriented and unilateral actions or ineffective habitual forms of practice. Self-emancipation is the key desired outcome of this examination as through this process nurses may become open to new models of practice. (Kim, 1999, p. 1209)

Whereas Taylor regarded each of her three types of reflection as having equal importance and thus selected depending on the situation, Kim's three phases of reflection form a developmental continuum along which practitioners can travel as they gradually extend their reflective abilities. In the 'descriptive phase', they are concerned primarily with building narratives of their practice through which they are able to 'open a door into the past'. The role of the facilitator at this stage is to stop the narrative from becoming too analytic and to ensure that it is, as far as possible, 'comprehensive and complete'. In the 'reflective phase', practitioners use those narratives to develop experiential knowledge and theory, and to begin to reflect on how that knowledge might be translated into action. The role of the facilitator in this phase is crucial, since Kim (1999) pointed out that it is extremely difficult for practitioners to be objective about their successes and failures in translating theory into action. Finally, the 'critical/emancipatory phase' involves a detailed critique of practice (where the term 'critique' is employed in Habermas' sense of the emancipation from self-deception through increased self-knowledge), which is ultimately a critique of the practitioners themselves.

We can see, then, that Kim's model sits somewhere between the epistemological and the ontological discourses of reflective practice discussed in the previous chapter, since it involves learning both about practice and about self. It could be argued that it shares many similarities with the framework developed by Chris Johns, for whom self exploration is the primary purpose of reflection, and for whom reflection must be guided by a facilitator.

Further reading

Kim's model of reflection is based on the work of the critical theorists (sometimes referred to collectively as the Frankfurt School) briefly referred to in Chapter 1. Under the leadership of Jürgen Habermas, critical theory developed initially out of Marxism and has a very overt agenda for social change through education. One of the earliest models of reflection based on critical theory came from the Marxist Paulo Freire (1972), who saw the reflective process as a means of identifying and freeing oneself from false consciousness, and ultimately as a revolutionary tool. This approach was further developed by educationalists such as Carr and Kemmis (1986), particularly in Chapter 5 of their book *Becoming Critical*; Mezirow (1981), who saw the outcome of reflection as being a 'perspective transformation'; and Stephen Brookfield (1995), for whom reflection involved uncovering and challenging the power structures that 'under-gird, frame, and distort educational processes and interactions'. It has also been used more recently as the framework for Beverley Taylor's (2006) work on reflective practice in nursing.

Kolb's model of reflexive learning

We will now examine a third model or methodology of reflection that attempts to integrate thinking and practice into a single act. This model is based on Kolb's cycle of experiential learning, which requires practitioners to actively experiment with their practice as part of the reflective cycle. We can see from Figure 3.3 that Kolb extends the reflective process beyond observation and reflection on past events by encouraging practitioners to theorize on their reflections and then to try out new approaches based on those theories. This, in turn, will result in new experiences, and so the cycle is repeated.

We suggested at the end of Chapter 2 that reflection offers the possibility of an alternative approach to practice in which knowing and doing are closely linked. The frameworks discussed above go some

Figure 3.3 Kolb's cycle of experiential learning

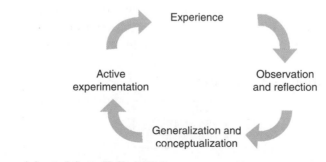

Source: Adapted from Kolb (1984).

way to fulfilling this promise by reversing the polarity between knowledge and practice and emphasizing knowledge *arising from* practice rather than knowledge *applied to* practice. This in turn elevates practitioners from technicians who apply knowledge produced by others into knowledge producers in their own right. However, thinking and doing are still presented as separate acts, where reflection is a mode of thought that enables learning from past practice to be applied to future practice.

By incorporating active experimentation into the model, Kolb has integrated thought and action so that neither makes sense without the other. The purpose of reflection is to formulate concepts and theories, and the purpose of theorizing is to generate hypotheses that can be tested once the practitioner is back in the practice setting. Depending on whether the hypotheses are confirmed or disproved, the practitioner will then begin the cycle anew by reflecting on the modified situation. Thus, whereas Dewey offers a model of *reflection* and Habermas offers a model of *reflective practice*, Kolb's model is truly *reflexive*.

Borton's framework

Borton (1970) took Kolb's model as the starting point for his framework and simplified it even further into three cue questions (Figure 3.4).

The first question that practitioners should ask themselves is a very simple and uncritical 'what?', which encourages them to describe the situation that they wish to reflect on. Borton's 'What?' stage is therefore based on Kolb's 'observation and reflection' stage. Second, they ask the question 'So what?', which prompts them to theorize from their description of the situation. This is based on Kolb's 'generalization and conceptualization' stage. Finally, they ask the question 'Now what?', which encourages them to plan an active intervention based on their theory, and which echoes Kolb's 'active experimentation' stage. Borton's framework is extremely stripped down and streamlined. This has the advantage of being very easy for practitioners to carry around in their heads, and is also eminently suitable for beginning reflective

Figure 3.4 Borton's reflective framework

```
• What?
• So what?
• Now what?
```

Source: Adapted from Borton (1970).

practitioners. However, due to its simple and minimal nature, it is best described through an example. In this example, a critical care nurse became very upset when a patient with whom she had formed a close relationship was deemed not suitable for resuscitation, and she disputed the consultant's decision in a heated discussion in front of the patient. She later reflected on how she had dealt with the situation by using Borton's framework.

What happened?

> I become very angry at the way in which the consultant took a life-and-death decision about this patient without any consultation with the staff who knew him best. I tried to put across my point of view, but she refused to listen. I eventually lost my temper and shouted at her in the middle of the ward. At this point, she stormed out.

This is the initial descriptive stage of the reflective process, in which the practitioner is reconstructing the situation from her own perspective. Reflection-on-action has sometimes been criticized for not being objective (Reece Jones, 1995; Bolton, 2005), but it is important that this descriptive reflective stage remains firmly in the subjective realm, since this provides the practitioner with the opportunity to explore her own personal emotions and perceptions of the situation. This descriptive reflection is eminently suitable for the novice, and even if the process terminates at this early stage, the practitioner will have been re-connected with her thoughts and feelings about the situation so that she can begin to learn from it.

So what am I to make of this?

> First, I shouldn't have lost my temper. The consultant probably felt just as uncomfortable as I did about the decision, and dealt with it by asserting her authority. Although I was right to feel angry, I shouldn't have reacted in the way I did. Perhaps I could have told the consultant how angry I was feeling rather than expressing my anger in front of the patient. She might have responded to rational argument, but by becoming angry, I simply gave her an excuse to storm out. I can see now that any chance of rational communication was blocked by our highly charged emotional states.

This second theory-building stage takes the practitioner beyond her earlier descriptive reflection, since she is not only reflecting on her thoughts and feelings, but learning from them. In the above example, the nurse is learning not only about the situation, but also about herself and (perhaps) about the consultant. Furthermore, she is beginning to develop a theory about how her reactions might have adversely influenced the situation, and about how she might have acted differently. Even if the process stops at this second stage, the nurse has achieved some valuable insights and is likely to behave differently the next time she encounters a similar situation.

Now what can I do to make the situation better?

> Now that I am feeling calmer, I think that I should make an appointment to see the consultant. We need to talk about the situation sensibly. I may not be able to change her mind, but I owe it to myself and to my patient to give it my best shot. I also need to let the consultant see that I am a professional practitioner and that my opinion counts for something.

Although the second stage was action-oriented in the sense that the practitioner might learn from the situation and act differently the next time it occurs, this final stage seeks to respond *reflexively* to the actual situation that is being reflected on. In the above example, the nurse has learnt not only to deal with the consultant differently in the future, but also attempts to resolve the ongoing problem in the light of her reflections on the situation.

Reflective moment

Now think of a situation from your own practice that you feel was left unresolved, and attempt to reflect on it by using Borton's three questions.

How useful did you find it? Which was the easiest question to answer? Which was the hardest? At which of Borton's stages do you usually reflect? Write down what you found most difficult about the process.

One of the problems with Borton's framework is that little attention is paid to the finer details of reflection. Although Borton offers a useful framework for structuring critical reflection at the macro level by suggesting a number of stages through which the focus of reflection-on-action might develop, he says little about the ways in which reflection might be conducted and facilitated within each stage of the process, that is, with the micro-structure of critical reflection. In the above example, the nurse is not prompted to explore particular issues specific to the situation, for example, inter-professional politics, decision-making, ethical theories or the legal rights of the patient.

Rolfe's framework

Gary Rolfe expanded Borton's framework by suggesting some cue questions for each stage (Rolfe et al., 2001). He also turned the final

Descriptive level of reflection	Theory- and knowledge-building level of reflection	Action-oriented (reflexive) level of reflection
What ...	**So what ...**	**Now what ...**
. . . is the problem/difficulty/reason for being stuck/reason for feeling bad/reason we don't get on/etc., etc.?	. . . does this tell me/teach me/imply/mean about me/my client/others/ our relationship/my client's care/the model of care I am using/my attitudes/my client's attitudes/etc., etc.?	. . . do I need to do in order to make things better/stop being stuck/improve my client's care/resolve the situation/feel better/get on better/etc., etc.?
. . . was my role in the situation?	. . . was going through my mind as I acted?	. . . broader issues need to be considered if this action is to be successful?
. . was I trying to achieve?	. . . did I base my actions on?	. . . might be the consequences of this action?
. . actions did I take?		
. . . was the response of others?	. . . other knowledge can bring to the situation?	
. . . were the consequences • for the client? • for myself? • for others?	• factual • practical • personal	
. . . feelings did it evoke • in the client? • in myself? • in others?	. . . could/should I have done to make it better? . . . is my new understanding of the situation?	
. . . was good/bad about the experience?	. . . broader issues arise from the situation?	

Figure 3.5 Rolfe's framework for reflexive practice

stage back on itself to form a reflexive cycle (Figure 3.5). You should note that this is a generic framework that can be employed to structure internal, spoken or written reflections either alone, with a facilitator, or in a group. As it is generic, it might not meet your specific needs, and the cue questions are therefore intended to be open to change and revision for different practitioners in different situations.

You will see from the arrows at the top of the framework in Figure 3.5 that it is both sequential and cyclical. In other words, it presents an ordered sequence of stages or levels, the last of which reflexively returns to the first. At the first level, practitioners initially reflect on the situation in order to describe it. They then reflect again at the second deeper level in order to construct personal theory and knowledge about the situation, that is, to learn from it. At the third level, they plan how they might improve the situation through their actions, reflecting on their consequences. However, their actions will hopefully bring about change, and so they then return to the initial descriptive level of reflection in order to work though the sequence again with the transformed situation. Furthermore, the cycles can continue until the situation is resolved. We will now explore each of the three levels in more detail and illustrate them with a Practice Focus.

Level 1: Descriptive reflection

As we noted earlier, some critics have pointed out that most practitioners do not reflect at these deeper levels, and that some will probably never progress further than the concrete thinking required for descriptive reflection. These novice reflective practitioners might therefore remain at the first level, at least until their thinking has developed sufficiently for them to be able to begin to construct personal knowledge and theory out of their experiences. Despite not progressing past the first level of reflection, these practitioners will nevertheless benefit from consciously considering their practice in a structured way, from thinking the process through, and from exploring their feelings and those of the other people involved in the incident.

Case example

What is the problem?
I am a social worker with a client who has difficulty relating to other people since his wife died nearly two years ago. He wishes to get out of the house more, but does not know how to go about it.

What was my role in the situation?
I felt that I needed to make things better for him by offering practical help and advice.
What was I trying to achieve?
I was trying to respond to the client's wishes by getting him more involved in the outside world.
What actions did I take?
I made practical suggestions, for example, to join clubs, take up evening classes, place an advertisement in the personal column of the local newspaper, etc. I even offered to accompany him to social events.
What was the response of others?
There were no others involved in the situation.

What were the consequences?
None of my suggestions worked, despite the client's best intentions.
What feelings did it invoke in the client? He said that he felt he had let me down.
What feelings did it invoke in me?
I felt as though I had failed him, and that my counselling skills were lacking.
What was good/bad about the experience?
I felt as though I had built a strong relationship with him. However, there were no positive outcomes despite our best efforts.

In this case example, it is important that the social worker begins to look at her own feelings and those of the client. Both parties seemed to be quite comfortable with the stalemate situation, which had been continuing for some time. It is only once the practitioner realizes that they both appear to be content to continue in a situation where each claims to be feeling bad, that she will be motivated to explore it further.

Level 2: Theory- and knowledge-building reflection

More advanced practitioners will find it beneficial to think not only about what happened, but also about *how* and *why* it happened; that is, about the underlying processes and dynamics of the situation. At this second level of reflection, they will be prompted to think not only about the theory and knowledge which they (perhaps unconsciously) applied to the situation, but what other knowledge and theory they *could* have applied. In other words, they will be encouraged to reflect on how the situation could have been handled differently.

Case example

So what does this tell me?
First, I need to accept the fact that we are getting nowhere, and that my counselling intervention does not appear to be very effective.

So what was going through my mind as I acted?
It is very difficult to recall exactly what I was thinking as I made suggestions to the client. Part of me seemed to realize that whatever I said would make no difference, but another part thought that this didn't really matter, as I was building a good therapeutic relationship with him.

So what did I base my actions on?
I thought at the time that I was following a model of counselling, but I can see now that perhaps I was acting in my own interest rather than the client's.

So what other knowledge can I bring to the situation?
My personal knowledge of this client suggests that he was very close to his wife, but that he didn't socialize very much, apart from with one or two close friends. My practical knowledge of similar situations tells me that I sometimes become stuck with clients and find it difficult to move forward. In one particular case, my manager suggested that I stopped working with the client. My factual knowledge tells me that this is not uncommon in counselling situations. The theory of transactional analysis suggests that we might be caught up in a 'game' in which each of us is getting a pay-off from failing to make progress with counselling. Some theorists also suggest that the counsellor should resist making direct suggestions to the client.

So what could I have done to make it better?
I should perhaps not have become so obsessed with trying to solve my client's problem for him. Perhaps it is not even the real problem.

So what is my new understanding of the situation?
Despite the fact that we appear to be making little or no progress, the client continues to want me to visit, so perhaps he is gaining something from it, even it if is not what we set out to achieve. Perhaps I am providing all the social contact that he needs, and so he is (perhaps unconsciously) deliberately ensuring that we continue with the counselling sessions by failing to make progress. On the other hand, perhaps my repeated failure to help him is giving him a (much needed) feeling of superiority over me. Perhaps it is also in my interest not to succeed with this client. It is possible that I find the sessions safe and comfortable, and that I am secretly worried

that if they are successful then I will have to move on to work with other less familiar clients.

So what broader issues arise from the situation?
I need to stop and reflect on my therapeutic relationships, and in particular, to consider whether I am really meeting my clients' needs. I was a little shocked when I realized that I have been here before with other clients. Perhaps I need more supervision with my counselling work.

The social worker appears to have learnt some important lessons from this second knowledge-building level of reflection. In particular, she has recognized a recurring pattern in her counselling work, and has made a decision to seek more supervision in order to prevent such difficulties from arising again. In some situations and for some practitioners, this will be as far as the reflective process can take them. Perhaps the situation has been resolved; perhaps it has moved on and it would be inappropriate to revisit it; or perhaps the practitioner does not have the autonomy or the authority to act on the situation. Even so, she will have learnt not only about herself and the way in which she dealt (or not) with the situation, but also how she might deal differently with similar situations when they next occur.

Level 3: Action-oriented (reflexive) reflection
However, in some cases the practitioner will have the opportunity to return to the situation with the intention of improving it, and this is where a reflexive framework for reflection-on-action can make its greatest contribution to practice.

Case example

Now what do I need to do in order to stop being stuck?
There are a number of ways that I could move this situation forward. If I am holding the client back, I could simply stop working with him and suggest that he is discharged. This action might give him a greater incentive to build up new and healthier relationships outside counselling. Alternatively, I could confront the client with my theory so that he also recognizes that we are stuck in a rut, or I could simply stop making suggestions to him and see how he reacts.

Now what broader issues need to be considered if this action is to be successful?
If the client is discharged, I need to consider alternative support mechanisms that are less likely to induce overreliance on the

system. If I confront him, I need to be prepared for his response, which is likely to be one of denial. Finally, if I simply stop making suggestions I will need to be prepared for criticism and rejection. Perhaps I need to talk to my supervisor in order to explore these options, and how I might handle them.

Now what might be the consequences of this action?
I would hope that the client might recognize that we have been playing games and move on. However, he might be unable or unwilling to accept the need for a change in our relationship and respond by demanding a different counsellor, or even by discharging himself. I also need to consider my own possible reaction to a change in our relationship, since I also appear to be gaining something from it.

In this case example, the social worker has a number of options that she can pursue, and clearly, her reflection is likely to have a direct impact on her practice. Furthermore, once the planning has taken place, the consequences of the action anticipated and thought through, and the action implemented, the practitioner will have to return to the descriptive level of reflection to consider the newly transformed situation in a true reflexive cycle.

Reflective moment

Return to the situation from your own practice that you reflected on earlier using Borton's three questions. Now repeat the exercise using the framework for reflexive practice that we have just outlined.

Once again, think about the following:

How useful did you find it? Which was the easiest level to reflect at? Which was the hardest? At which level do you usually reflect? Did the addition of the cue questions to Borton's model make it easier or more difficult to use? Why?

We have, up until now, focussed entirely on what Schön (1983) referred to as reflection-on-action, that is, on retrospectively reflecting on our practice after and away from the event. However, Schön argued that more advanced practitioners also reflect *in* action, that is, during and as part of their practice. We can perhaps see how Rolfe's framework could be used to reflect-in-action by formulating and testing out questions and theories in real time as the situation unfolds. In the above example, the social worker might then have reflected on some of her ideas and put them into practice while she was still with the client rather than afterwards. Schön (1983) referred to this process of theorizing and testing ideas during practice as 'on-the-spot-experimenting' or 'knowing-in-action', in which the practitioner 'becomes a researcher in the practice context'. Reflection-in-action will be discussed in detail in Chapter 8.

Conclusion

This chapter has argued that, in order to compete as a viable alternative to technical rationality, the reflective paradigm requires some structure in the form of methodologies and methods, or what reflective practitioners often refer to as models and frameworks. We examined three models of reflection and some associated frameworks, based on the philosophies of John Dewey, Jürgen Habermas and Donald Kolb respectively. We suggested that whereas Dewey offered a model of reflection and Habermas offered a model of reflective practice, Kolb's model was truly reflexive in linking thought back to action in a single process. We therefore gave most attention to the frameworks based on Kolb's model, particularly those offered by Borton and Rolfe. We ended with the suggestion that these reflexive frameworks could also be applied to practice in real time as a form of reflection-in-action.

Reflective moment

Now turn back to the aims which you identified at the start of the chapter. To what extent have they been met? Write a paragraph outlining the factual and practical knowledge you have acquired through reading this chapter and doing the exercises. Write a second paragraph identifying any aims which you feel were only partially met or not met at all. As in previous chapters, divide your page into three columns. Head the first column 'What I need to learn', and make a list of any outstanding issues which you would like to learn more about. For example, you might wish to find out more about critical theory. Head the second column 'How I will learn it', and write down the ways in which your learning needs could be addressed; for example, through further reading, through attending study days, or through talking to other people. Head the third column 'How I will know that I have learnt it', and try to identify how you will know when you have met your needs.

4

Understanding reflective writing

Melanie Jasper

Introduction

Since the first edition of this book we have seen the growth and accommodation of reflective writing as a learning strategy within professional education across the disciplines. There is a growing awareness of the personalized and individualized knowledge located within practice that needs individual exploration and articulation before it finds a voice and dissemination to a wider audience, and an acceptance that a vehicle for exploring and understanding that unique nature of practice is through reflective activity, often in a written form. However, writing, by its very nature, is an individual activity, and located within the subjectivity of experience of the writer as a person, rendering it a perfect medium for moving from reflective analysis of an experience to critical reflexivity located within the person's socially constructed reality.

A requirement for reflective writing of some sort is now embedded in all pre-registration preparation for practice in health and social care disciplines. There are numerous examples of student doctors, radiographers, occupational therapists, physiotherapists, social workers and nurses learning their craft through reflections on their experiences in practice (see Guide to further reading). Indeed, assessment of reflective writing has become commonplace as a means to verify the achievement of competence in practice arenas. Writing at this level tends to be descriptive and documentary, demonstrating beginning skills in reflective learning which are later honed and developed once registration with a professional body is recorded and post-registration development in practice begins to occur. We now see evidence of the growth and valuing of reflective analysis in written forms through strategies for continuing professional development, whether or not these are within formal educational programmes (Orland-Barak, 2005; Bolton, 2006; Chirema, 2007). Reflection following initial professional education is more likely to focus on an understanding and development of the reflector through grappling with challenges in their practice, and to adopt a more critical and meta-cognitive approach as practitioners attempt to make sense of and learn from the experiences in practice. This suggests a growing awareness of the differences between reflective analysis and critical reflection, and that the latter arises as practitioners develop their own skills, knowledge and expertise as a result of individualized practice and experience.

Furthermore, Shapiro, Kasman and Shafer (2006) suggest that reflective writing helps to nurture characteristics in practitioners such as narrative competence, empathy, emotional equilibrium, self-healing capacity and well-being, which are less amenable to development from the traditional logical-rationalist educational strategies characterized within many healthcare professionals' initial education. Certainly, self-awareness and agency are usually the result of reflective activity.

Alongside this personal growth and development, post-qualification starts to take on a more critical stance as the practitioner gains the confidence in their practice environment to evaluate and challenge the assumptions and socio-political contexts that drive healthcare delivery. The deeper and more sophisticated reflective activity seen at this level often results in consequences beyond the individual practitioner, such as practice change and development, or even fundamental challenges to organizational culture. As a result, the products of critical reflection are contributing to professional as well as personal development, whether at the level of the individual practitioner, within clinical environments or wider in terms of how practitioners are utilized and deployed within a service. Our understanding of the mechanisms and processes involved in reflective writing has also grown over the past decade. Indeed, we did question, when planning the revision of this book, whether a chapter on reflective writing was still necessary. However, while the primary purpose of this chapter was originally to help the tentative writer take the first steps in developing confidence to write reflectively, it is clear that help in writing at the higher reflective, analytical and critical levels is much needed to enable practitioners to explore and understand fully the hidden nuances of practice and the assumptions that guide that practice. We have therefore expanded the original chapter into two; this first chapter concentrates on exploring how critical reflection can be developed through the process of reflective writing. We will discuss what we mean by reflective writing and explore how writing in itself can be seen as a process for learning; we will look at some of the barriers to writing and how these can be overcome. The next chapter explores techniques and strategies for critical reflective writing in the practice context and in particular, considers the ways in which writing may help us to develop critical thinking skills and lead to knowledge creation.

Considering reflective writing

In the first three chapters of this book you have been invited to engage in 'reflective writing' exercises. You have probably looked at these, picked up a pencil and tackled the exercises (or not!), but did you actually stop to think about the *processes* behind what we have been asking you to do, and why, or have you simply engaged in the writing as learning exercises without considering that the act of writing itself may well be enabling you to learn?

We discuss many different strategies and approaches to critical reflection in this book, from individual contemplative reflection, to reflection with others; from structured reflection through various different models, to reflection as a research strategy for uncovering knowledge. In this chapter we explore the value of written reflection, that is, of deliberately using strategies of writing as a way of reflecting and as a way of learning from our experience. Writing can, of course, be used together with any of the strategies discussed in other chapters; what we hope to establish here is the added value that can be gained when you decide to write reflectively as well as, or in addition to, verbal and contemplative reflection.

People often ask us 'why write?' There seems to be a widespread reluctance among clinical practitioners to create written records of the ways they practice, let alone writing about practice as a way of reflecting and learning from it. Much of this reluctance arises from the fundamental way of working of most practitioners: by our very nature and self-definition we are 'doers', we act out our professionalism by doing a job. Our primary form of communicating with others is verbal: we talk to each other, we talk to our patients, clients and families. This verbal communication is part of the way in which we practice; it is very often embedded within the culture of our practice and so we are usually comfortable with our verbal skills. We are practitioners as a result of practicing. Why, then, do we need to write about it? What is the purpose and what may we get out of it?

The aims of this chapter are:

1. to explore the nature of reflective writing;
2. to explore the ways that reflective writing is used and to look at the benefits of reflective writing as a learning tool;
3. to enable you to understand your own attitude and relationship to writing; and
4. to introduce the concept of critical thinking as part of critical reflection.

Reflective moment

Think carefully about our aims for Chapter 4. Now think about your own practice and how these aims might contribute towards developing it.

Based on our aims above, identify and write down some of your own, both in terms of what you hope to know and what you hope to be able to do after reading Chapter 4. We will return to these at the end of the chapter.

What is *reflective* writing?

In using the term *reflective writing*, we are referring to the processes involved in writing that can be utilized as means in themselves to help us learn from our experiences. Thus, reflective writing involves engaging in and completing the reflective cycle using the processes of writing as an instrument to help you learn. Reflective writing, in this context, differs from other forms of writing only in that it has one primary purpose: it is undertaken for the specific purpose of learning; to enable us to come to a different, or deeper, understanding of whatever we are reflecting on. Thus, using a model of reflection such as those to be found in this book, or using some other sort of strategy which enables you to describe, analyze and evaluate your experiences and to write them down, is useful (some would argue essential) in helping you to write reflectively.

This essential feature of reflective writing is often overlooked when we start on the process, which may explain why many of us find it difficult to write reflectively. Much of the advice given by educators, in journal articles and even by professional bodies, tends to focus on the descriptive and emotional stages of reflective writing without sufficient emphasis being placed on the evaluative and restorative elements, or those that help you take a critical stance within the practice context. As a result, many people have been disillusioned by their experiences of written exercises such as critical incident analyses or reflective journals, because the links between the components of the experience and the learning to be achieved are not made. Many others have been put off reflective writing as a result of rules being externally imposed, concerning *what* you are expected to write about, and *how* you are supposed to write it; requirements to 'bare your soul' and make public what you would prefer to keep private; and the worries about writing things down that may have professional consequences, such as exploring instances of malpractice, naming clients and colleagues, or drawing attention to deficits in care.

For reflective writing to serve the purpose of helping you to learn, it is vital that you set the parameters or rules for the writing and that you are in control of the whole process. Any writing you do in this way needs to satisfy the purposes that you want to use it for, and not be influenced by the needs of others. Part of being successful as a reflective writer is that you are able to select from the array of models and structures available, or even create your own strategies, and that you feel comfortable with what you are writing and have control over who sees it. Also, part of this is that you control the product of the writing; it is up to you to decide who, if anybody, sees your writing, and no-one can force you to make public what you have written. Your first ventures into reflective writing may have been to satisfy requirements for courses or for portfolio completion. Despite the interpretations that are often put on these, neither dictates the content of your writing; you can make choices as to what to use in illustration or evidence that you have achieved the requirements of, for instance, learning outcomes or criteria for the professional body.

Thus, the success of writing reflectively, as with any other reflective activity that you will meet in this book, is in completing the reflective cycle. It is often neither the subject nor the content of what you reflect on that is necessarily important, but its analysis in terms of what can be drawn out in understanding the assumptions on which it is based, and the learning that occurs as a result. We see reflective writing as one way of doing this, as one tool in the kit bag, which will suit some people and not others, just as many of the techniques throughout the book will have more appeal to some of us than others. This suggests that there is something different involved in the process of writing things down; something that will not happen if reflection remains verbal or within our head. Understanding the nature of reflective writing helps us to overcome any reluctance to use it within our practice, so we'd like to take some time to explore your understanding of your own attitude and feelings about writing.

We have seen that the very act of writing is thought by many to be a learning activity in its own right. However, for some of us, unless we have taken the time to think about it, our experiences of writing are locked into our past educational experiences or our need to write within the confines expected in our professional role: we learnt to write for other people, and we write *what* others want us to write in the *style* others expect. For example, think of the difference between writing an academic essay and writing a letter to a friend. In other words, we *learn-to-write* through the processes of socialization and teaching. We learn the externally imposed rules of writing for other people, which are not necessarily, and in fact are often the complete opposite of, the notion of *writing-to-learn*, which is at the heart of reflective writing.

Reflective moment

Think back to the last time that you decided to write about something – it may have been a letter, a shopping list, a report for work, some client records, or even an academic piece of work. Draw a line down the middle of your page. On the left hand side, try to answer the following questions:

1. What did you write?
2. What was the purpose (why did you write it)?
3. How did you decide what, and what not, to write?
4. How did you decide on the order of what you wrote?
5. How did you organize or structure what you wrote?

On the right-hand side of the page, try to think about the 'why' questions – why were you writing, and why did you include some things and leave others out? Why did you order it in this way? Why did you organize what you were writing in this way?

Now, try to think a bit deeper about the process of writing itself and why you decided to write rather than commit to memory. Did the act of writing as a mental activity enable other things to happen? For instance, if writing a shopping list, did you remember, for some reason, other things to add to your list that you weren't intending to get or which you had 'forgotten'? If you were writing a report on a client, did you start to make connections between things that you hadn't previously seen before?

We will ask you to use your answers to this exercise as we work through the rest of the chapter.

Two concepts, identified by Allen, Bowers and Diekelmann (1989) as *learning-to-write* and *writing-to-learn,* can be seen as fundamental to why many of us do not see the value of writing reflectively. Many of our previous experiences of writing have probably been rooted in providing some sort of evidence to others that we have learnt something,

Table 4.1 A comparison of the assumptions of the two concepts learning to write and writing to learn

Learning to write	Writing to learn
Students can successfully learn content whether or not they can write well	Writing is a process through which content is learned or understood (as opposed to memorized or reported)
Writing and thinking involve different skills. Each can, and perhaps should, be taught separately	Writing skills are primarily thinking skills (competence in one is inseparable from competence in the other)
Knowing something is logically prior to writing about it	Writing is a process of developing an understanding or coming to know something
Writing is a sequential, linear activity which involves the cumulative mastery of components like sentence construction or outlining	Writing is a dialectical, recursive process rather than linear or sequential
Communication is the main purpose of writing. Written work is a product in which the student reports what he or she already knows	Higher order conceptual skills can only evolve through a writing process in which the writer engages in an active, on-going dialogue with him or herself and others. Learning and discovery are purposes as important for writing as communication
The student's audience is most often assumed to be the instructor	Different disciplines utilize different conceptual processes and thus have different standards for writing. Students can best learn writing within their own disciplines while writing for real, concrete audiences

Source: Adapted from Allen, Bowers and Diekelmann (1989, p. 7).

as opposed to the process being useful to us personally in helping us to understand through a creative process of writing for ourselves. Table 4.1 shows the features of these two concepts, and further exploration of them may help us to understand in more depth just why the idea of writing is so difficult for some of us to embrace.

The chances are that your past experiences of writing, at least throughout your formal education, are located within the *learning-to-write* framework. On the whole, we wrote what we thought others wanted us to write. For instance, we would re-write from textbooks in order to show a teacher that we had read (but not necessarily under-stood or learnt) the material; or we would write an exam paper or essay which yet again involved a repetition of theory or knowledge, to prove that we could remember it. At times you may have written an essay asking you to discuss ideas, or analyze, or even be creative, but this is most likely still to have been at someone else's instigation rather than defined by you. Moreover, your success would have been dependent upon you correctly decoding the unseen rules about what was being asked of you. For example, how many times have you slaved over an essay, only to have it returned with a disappointing grade and the comment 'You haven't answered the question'? The main assumption of this concept is that thinking and writing are essentially different, and indeed, that writing is a means to an end, not the end in itself.

You will also have been 'taught' the rules of writing as a formal process for communication. These rules become so ingrained that it is difficult for us to conceive of writing that we can understand if it doesn't follow them. This is illustrated when we are faced with writing in languages which are not our own, or in media that are different from our usual way of working, such as poetry or metaphor. Not only are we taught what to write, but also how to write it, and the writing therefore becomes the medium for communication, but not the message. As a byproduct of this, we gain ideas about writing being right or wrong which influence us throughout our lives. This idea of writing as right or wrong is amazingly persistent for most people, and acts as a barrier for us when attempting to start writing reflectively. If your only writing has ever been for public consumption, and if this has been judged in some way, then it is difficult to conceive of taking control of that writing and seeing it as value free, that it is by you, for you, and that no-one else's judgement matters. In our work as educationalists and facilitators of reflective writing, one of our most challenging tasks is helping people to overcome the anxiety that makes them ask 'Am I doing it right?', or 'Is this what you want?'

Reflective moment

Think back to your schooldays. Try to describe to a colleague, or write down, your attitude to writing as a child. Why did you write? Who did you write for? How did you learn what was 'right' and 'wrong' about your writing? Think about the messages that your childhood experiences have given you about the value and purpose of writing that you have carried with you into your adult life.

Now think about your professional education. Did this reinforce those previous experiences of writing, or enable you to develop different skills? Discuss this with your colleague.

What is your attitude to writing now?

Reconceptualizing writing

The right-hand side of Table 4.1 proposes a different concept of writing, one where the process of writing in itself is a seen as a way of learning. The assumptions underpinning this concept are that writing and thinking go hand in hand, that writing evolves from thinking, and that creativity arises from thinking about and doing writing. Furthermore, it is suggested that understanding comes from writing, that we learn as a result of interacting with the subject matter, and that in the process, this material becomes transformed into 'knowing'. Thus, the very process of writing is not seen as a passive activity directed by others, but is in itself dynamic, leading to new connections being made and new understanding occurring.

The last three features in the table are particularly important to our concept of reflective writing, in that they acknowledge the individual nature of writing for the person. In effect, they lift writing above the basic idea of writing for others, and transform it into a way through which we can combine thinking and writing in a dialogue with ourselves and others, and to develop our own understanding and create knowledge out of our experience.

Now look back to what you wrote in your reflections on the last piece of writing that you did. The last questions asked were to help you to think about what happened as a result of the process of writing; whether you added something to your shopping list that was not previously there, or whether you began to see something in a different light as a result of writing the incident down. This provides an illustration of the *transformative* nature of writing when viewed from the *writing-to-*

learn perspective; the act of writing in itself adds to the way in which we view our experiences. So, to return to our earlier question: *What is it about writing that adds something to our reflective processes?*

Features of writing

Writing as a purposeful activity

First, writing is a purposeful activity. We always write for some purpose, even if it is simply a note for the milkman. Moreover, it is impossible to concentrate on writing while trying to do something else. As a result, we have to give the whole of our attention to writing; no other thoughts can be going on in our heads at the same time other than very simple things such as 'Do I need another cup of coffee?' The combination of thinking and translating those thoughts into writing involves complex mental and physical processes that force us to focus on the task in hand. In order to do this, we need to dedicate special time to writing, and for some of us this involves almost ritualistic behaviour, such as having to have our writing space organized in a particular way, having completed certain other tasks before sitting down to write, or even simply a matter of having the right number of pencils or our favourite pen.

Many of us have now abandoned pens and paper in favour of computers and hand-held devices that bring with them their own capacity for idiosyncrasy – for instance, the authors of this book each admit to different ways of 'having' to write in a particular way on screen, whether that be formatting and correcting as they write, or splurging everything out regardless, then going back to correct later. New rituals grow, in the same ways that we became familiar with hand writing, that enable us to be comfortable with the techniques of writing and for these to satisfy our need for safety and security. New skills also have to be learnt when encompassing the new technologies – typing skills such as whether you can touch type and watch the screen while typing or relying on the two-fingered method, affect how you can write and record what you want to write. Similarly, the capacity to 'cut and paste' or to edit in progress all affect the very ways in which we 'write' and reconfigure as we go along. We no longer have to rub pencil out, or cross inked words from the text – instead, *highlight and delete* removes the thoughts as though they were never there.

The consequences of all these factors are that when we write, we make a commitment to both the content and process of what we are writing. When writing reflectively, this commitment becomes all important, in that we need a stimulus or a purpose for doing it, and very often this arises from within ourselves and our practice.

Writing as a way of ordering our thoughts

Second, writing forces us to impose some sort of order to the content of what we are writing. However, this order needs only to make sense to ourselves; it does not have to be an imposed order acceptable to others unless we are deliberately writing for an audience, such as an essay, a book chapter, or a piece of work for which we have a definite structure. This notion of order for writing is often quite intimidating, and for some it is complete anathema and inhibits them from writing because yet again there is a fear of getting it 'wrong'. However, if we try to put aside the notion of a 'received' order that will please someone else, and think instead about what our own needs are, we can see that we always have some sort of order to what we write, even if we do not consciously decide on it initially.

Return again to your answers to the questions about the last time you wrote. You will probably be able to see that, quite unconsciously at the time, you wrote with a clearly defined purpose, and that you imposed an order on what you were writing. Where did this order come from? Did it just happen, or did you make decisions about how to structure your writing? While a structure might well appear out of the ether, it is more likely that you were responding to some internal rules that made sense to you, or that have arisen as a result of your previous experiences, and that help you to feel comfortable with your writing.

The process of writing not only helps us to find a structure for its content, but in choosing an order to the points, it helps us to prioritize and identify what is important and what is not of such significance. This happens because the speed of our writing is limited to the speed at which we can record our thoughts. This slows us down, and we go through a process of mentally sifting and pulling out what we feel are the most important things to capture in writing. We cannot write at the speed at which we think, or even at the speed at which we talk, and so writing reflectively is going to be very different in content and structure to the way that we reflect when talking to others or contemplatively to ourselves. In fact, this has three distinct advantages.

First, in writing things down we are forced to acknowledge issues that may be ignored if we are carrying on a conversation or reflecting inside our heads. Second, we can put a hierarchical order to issues that are significant to us, rather than to how they are seen by other people. Third, this enables us to work through these issues as we have identified them, rather than being sidetracked away to other things. These make reflective writing an extremely personal process and one which, unlike contemplative writing where we may get stuck going round and round in circles in our head, enables us to work systematically through a process of reflection.

Writing as a permanent record

This leads us to the third feature of writing that distinguishes it as a reflective strategy: writing creates a permanent record that can be returned to and reconsidered. Why is this important? The act of writing helps us to remember things, not only those which we think we have forgotten, but also things that may be hidden or overlaid by others which take priority. In trying to recall things that have happened to us and recount them verbally, we are selective in what we remember. This is the problem of hindsight bias, for which other forms of reflection have sometimes been criticized. Very often we are convinced that we have remembered every detail, yet others who were also there at the time might say 'Yes, but do you remember...too?', thereby jogging our memory and filling in another piece of the picture. Think, too, about the times that you have tried to teach someone else to do something; a skill, or even some theoretical knowledge. It is often only when you try to explain something to another person that you realize whether you really know it or not. In writing things down, we record what our memory allows us to remember at the time. This might be close to the event, or at some time distant, and creates at least one account of the event that can be used in the future for reflective activity. This original description can act as a memory jogger the next time you read it, when more or different details and explanations of what has happened occur to us. As a result of the time and space created, we are often able to take a different perspective on the event and see it in a different way by filling in more information, or considering it in the light of new or alternative experiences and knowledge. In terms of taking a *critical* approach to reflection, this capacity to consider events from different contexts, such as within a policy or financial context, and individualizing the content of the event in relation to the assumptions we made about it, is crucial in the learning process and in developing alternative understandings.

The four excerpts which follow come from a student's reflective review of her experiences in a supervision group over a period of two and a half years. The first was written when the group had only been together for a short time, and the last excerpt presents a view of where her experiences of the group have taken her in terms of her learning about herself.

Excerpt one:

The first clinical supervision session was unfortunate. There were comments passed during this, what could be termed as a psychological experiment, which culminated in an hour of uncomfortable silence interspersed with two of us asking for structure and being told by other members that we were trying to control. Since then, the meetings have been somewhat stilted and awkward but I will wait and see what transpires next semester. There certainly has not been any learning achieved yet. A new Learning Outcome for semester two is to critically explore models and beliefs regarding supervision thereby realizing its relevance to my learning from this course.

Excerpt two:

Unfortunately the group dynamics remain rather difficult within the supervision groups with two who are controlling, one who wishes structure but is being told she is controlling, one who views us all with what would appear to be disdain, and others who try to contribute but with little enthusiasm. I am afraid I remain in the latter group. I find difficulties in attending for that hour with work commitments and often arrive tense and rushed. I am trying to change my beliefs regarding the group but by the time I have recovered from the rush to attend and have settled in, the time has passed and the end leaves me feeling the same way. The atmosphere for me does not encourage the in-depth reflection and analysis I was hoping for; however, I am beginning to realize what a powerful tool for clinical practice this style of supervision could be.

Excerpt three:

The supervision group has remained unhelpful, however one member had expressed the desire to leave the course. Due to this four of us decided to meet fortnightly to give her and ourselves support and encouragement in completing the assignments. It was interesting to meet in such a forum where all of us felt that we should have taken more responsibility to change the structure of the group instead of playing the victims. I now realize the power and support that such a group can bring where the environment feels safe. Although the meetings were dedicated to academic achievement rather than practical issues, it could be seen how that type of meeting would be uniquely powerful in supporting practitioners to reflect and analyze practice.

Excerpt four:

Over the last four semesters there has been learning; however, it has not always been achieved in the way I was expecting. What did have an enormous impact on me was the Practice Development through Supervision unit. I have learnt so much from writing the assessment concerning my contribution to the group, and what started out as very negative has become a learning experience. The supervision assignment highlights how what I believed was an equivocal experience due to other people's attitudes and beliefs, actually was failing to realize that I had just as much responsibility as other members of the group to make the sessions work for all of us. It is always easy to blame other people when things go wrong, which often occurs in professional practice. The sessions made me realize the importance of understanding other people's perspectives. I do not perceive that the supervision sessions were anything other than dire, yet they made me realize the need for that model in professional practice. Due to the unfortunate group dynamics, I did not utilize the groups for any of my experiences in clinical or educational practice, but the importance for structured reflection in practice was obvious to me through the meetings that other practitioners have their own points of view which should be aired if a cohesive team is hoped for. Changes in practice to evidence-based and effective practice can only come about when each professional from each profession acknowledges each other equally. The supervision group was made up of specialists from different fields and each had a different perspective, but it was clear that after all we are all wishing to provide the same high-quality service to people in our care... With the poor group dynamics and the frustration with the clinical supervision groups, I became a victim rather than taking the responsibility to ask for help and take control of my own education. This has resulted in a lot of wasted opportunities for learning and for the support that I craved.

The permanent record illustrated in these extracts, written incrementally as an experience developed over time, illustrates how we can look back and learn from events in the past. Of course, we are able to do this at any time by mentally recalling events; however, what these excerpts show quite clearly is that this person's perspective on the experiences actually changes over time, and it is unlikely that this observation can occur if contemporaneous records are not made at the time that the events are unfolding. It is easy to reconsider with hindsight, and certainly this student can put her experiences of the past into the perspective of the present. However, what she would have omitted if she had not written as she went along were the features of the experience that are no longer significant in the present. By writing them down, she can reflect on how the totality of the experience has brought her to her current ways of understanding the learning that has been achieved. Perhaps one of the most important points to make here is that the past cannot be changed, and our reactions and perceptions of it at the time were what was significant and important to that person at the time, and was their reality of the situation. By engaging in critical reflection over a period of two years, this student was able to accept the uncomfortable feelings that she had as part of the learning she went through, and even comes to value them as essential in turning something that she considered as negative at the time into a positive event for learning for her present and the future.

In writing, we allow ourselves the time to put things aside and return to them when we are ready to deal with them. We 'capture the moment' and can then return to it at our leisure. One student, who had started to use reflective writing on his computer to help him work through difficult issues at work, said that an advantage in writing things down was that it made him deal with them, unlike being able to ignore them if they were in his head. He said that once they had appeared on paper there was a constant reminder, and this acted as a prompt to sort them out, and that to some extent this was a hidden effect of writing; it acts as a conscience so that you cannot conveniently forget things; indeed, that they may turn out to be the key to a problem that you have not yet found.

Writing as a way of making connections between ideas

The process of writing can, in itself, be seen as a creative one. Very often, we sit down with the intention of writing one thing, with a plan of some sort, and end up with something different from what we had envisaged. Our mind takes us down certain paths as a result of considering the material in front of us at that particular time, and it helps us to make an alternative, and sometimes unexpected, sense of what we are seeing. Thus, we may make connections between pieces of information that in the past we had not contemplated. The writing process helps us to *integrate* disparate information-sets into new combinations, enabling us to take a different perspective on an issue. These four features of writing are summarized in Table 4.2.

Table 4.2 Summary of the features of writing

Writing as a purposeful activity	Writing as a way of ordering our thoughts	Writing as a permanent record	Writing as a way of making connections between ideas
• Provides a focus for thinking about an issue • Sharpens our focus or explicitness of ideas through deliberate word choice • Identifies key or important points • The active nature of writing promotes critical thinking • Interacting with material is a key variable in learning from writing	• Creates an order that is logical to us • Helps to stop chaotic thinking • Identifies priorities • Identifies multiple elements of the issues • Helps us to sort out what is important from what is not • Aids understanding by analysis • Aids development of critical thinking	• It 'captures' the moment • Helps us not to forget important elements of an experience • Allows time for contemplation • Allows perspective to change over time • Allows reflection and consideration	• Gives a rounded picture • Helps to integrate previously separate and unconnected pieces of information • Helps to integrate theory with practice • Aids personal insight • Helps us to see things differently • Helps frame action

Bringing the 'critical' into written reflection

As we saw earlier, the reflective writing process is a way of making connections between previously disparate pieces of information, of developing ways of organizing or reorganizing thoughts, and of exploring issues and structures so as to be able to take a new perspective on them. As you will have understood from the preceding chapters, we can reflect at different levels and with different outcomes and results for our understanding of issues and events. At advanced and expert levels of practice it would be expected that practitioners are reflecting in sophisticated and 'critical' ways that move far beyond the descriptive levels of reflection seen in beginning practice. In fact, any educational activity taken at Masters level or above would have an expectation of reflective activity that meets the criteria imposed by educational institutions for awards at that level. Yet much of the published work in the past decade suggests that practitioners are not achieving the higher levels of reflective activity that we would expect to see (Brodie, 2007; Chirema, 2007). This suggests that further work needs to be done in enabling practitioners to understand the nature of critical thinking, and thus critical reflection, in order for them to be able to utilize reflective writing in the sophisticated way envisaged.

Brunt (2005) suggests that 'critical' reflection facilitates an understanding of one's own perception of the situation, as well as an examination of the underlying assumptions. Indeed, many writers see the reflective process as key to developing critical thinking, and reflective writing in some form as a crucial process of enabling it to happen. Critical thinking is regarded as one of the ways that practitioners make decisions about their practice, and developing the ability to think critically is now an essential component in the majority of educational programmes.

What do we mean by critical thinking? Critical thinking has been defined as: 'The process of purposeful, self-regulatory judgement; an interactive reflective, reasoning process' (Facione, Facione and Sanchez, 1994, p. 345).

Despite the brevity of this definition, critical thinking is recognized as a complicated, complex and intricate process that involves problem-solving, reasoning in considering opposing viewpoints or competing theories, and an attitude of inquiry. Ennis (1985) suggests that in addition to these processes, critical thinking also involves making decisions related to how to act or to believe. Table 4.3 summarizes the characteristics of a critical thinker identified by the American Philosophical Association (Facione, 1990) and Brookfield (1987).

In short, critical thinking is about weighing up all the possibilities for action and being able to make a reasoned and rational choice. Kintgen Andrews (1991) suggests further that critical thinking is a process of meta-cognition, of thinking about thinking, while Paul suggests that the practice of *dialogical* reasoning: 'plots two or more opposing points of view in competition with each other. Support for each view, and the raising and countering of objections, is integral to the process' (Paul, 1996, cited by Boychuk Duchscher, 1999).

Table 4.3 Features of a critical thinker

The ideal critical thinker is	Critical thinkers are people
• habitually inquisitive	• engaging in productive and positive activity
• well-informed	
• trustful of reason	• viewing their thinking as a process rather than an outcome
• open-minded	
• honest in facing personal biases	• varying in their manifestations of critical thinking according to context
• prudent in making judgements	
• willing to reconsider	• experiencing triggers to critical thinking as positive or negative
• clear about issues	
• diligent in seeking relevant information	• feeling comfortable with the emotive as well as the rational elements of the critical thinking process
• orderly in complex matters	
• reasonable in the selection of criteria	(after Brookfield, 1987)
• focused in inquiry	
• persistent in seeking results which are as precise as the subject and the circumstances of inquiry permit	
(after Facione, 1990)	

Sources: Adapted from Facione (1990) and Brookfield (1987).

Reflective moment

When looking at the criteria in Table 4.3, it is easy to assume that we all possess them. However, it can be an illuminating experience to attempt to assess oneself against these criteria, and to provide evidence, in the form of examples, of how you could demonstrate to someone else that you practice as a critical thinker. You may like to include this exercise as an entry in your portfolio.

The components of critical thinking have been identified by Brookfield (1987) as:

• *Identifying and challenging assumptions:* This means ensuring that you write down the assumptions that you made in relation to an event that you describe. These assumptions may be the knowledge or theory that you used, particular paradigm cases that you can remember, or experiential learning. You may like to think more widely about the nature of the assumptions underpinning the event, such as your beliefs and values about the role of patients in their own care; about your role in the power relationship you have with people as a professional; or perhaps even the political or economic circumstances that result in decisions about the availability of alternatives for care packages for different types of clients. In addition, you may be using information from your client or their family, written records, or verbal clues that have been passed on by others. Remember to consider what you take in through your senses: what you see, smell, feel by touch or hear. Perhaps there was an emotional reaction or component to the event that also contributes to your perception of the situation. The description of events that you make needs to be as accurate a record of what happened as possible so that you can identify the assumptions that you made.

When exploring an experience reflectively, it is worth, in attempting to be critical, identifying the assumptions on which each of your actions are based. For instance, in choosing one form of therapeutic intervention over another, ask yourself what influenced your decision – evidence of efficacy, government recommendations, previous experience with another client, cost, protocol or procedure, direction from another colleague? Then, try to think outside of this box of assumptions and test out for yourself what may have been the consequences of working from different assumptions to the ones that influenced you in the first place.

- *Recognizing the importance of context:* Our actions are never context-free; we all work within the confines of our experiences of the world, time and the places where we have lived. These ultimately interfere with and affect the way that we see others. Exploring the context of events and acknowledging the limitations of our perceptions enables us to think more analytically, and therefore critically. Writing these down provides us with a way of objectifying our experiences; we are able to stand outside the experiences as personal and view them from a different perspective.

- *Exploring and imagining alternatives:* Critical thinking involves being able to compare and evaluate different solutions to problems or to consider events in order to uncover new and different ways of perceiving the world. Brookfield (1987, p.18) suggests that this involves:

coming to realise that every belief we hold, every behaviour we cherish as normal, every social or economic arrangement we perceive as fixed and unalterable can be and is regarded by others as bizarre, inexplicable, and wholly irrational.

- It is salutary to remember that other people will not 'see' things and events in the same way that you do. Two people will rarely give the same description of an event, even if they were standing next to each other when it happened. Hence, features of an event that you see as important or significant may not be the same for other people. This is understandable when you set each person's perception within the context of her own life experiences. Writing enables us to explore and imagine alternative viewpoints by providing us with structures and questions which challenge our previous way of looking at things.

- *Reflective scepticism*
Being sceptical protects us from accepting 'universal truths' or that there is only ever one explanation for an event or one way of looking at it. Developing scepticism leads us to question and seek alternative answers, and may lead ultimately to the development of new understandings by encouraging us to reject previously accepted explanations.

The concept of critical thinking can be developed through writing by overtly using these components as a check list, and by auditing our entries against them. In turn, this may well lead on to *creative* thinking, where not only can we justify and defend our actions, but we may also develop new understandings and perspectives on a situation, or come to understand a past event in a different light. As one nurse in Jasper's (1999) study said:

> I think creative thinking is actually taking the bits of knowledge that you already have and producing something entirely new from that; that you come forward from what you already know. I think you develop by recognising the infinite combinations of little bits of knowledge, little pockets of knowledge.

The processes of writing discussed earlier in this chapter, the need to create a space for writing and to treat it as a deliberative activity, provide the mechanisms for facilitating the development of critical thinking. The physical activity of structuring and restructuring or seeking explanations and new ways of knowing, leads us to look for unique explanations in themselves that may direct action and affect outcomes for our clients.

Conclusion

The aim of this chapter was to explore the nature of reflective writing and present it as an essential component of critical reflection. In presenting reflective writing as a type of writing that is under the control and direction of the writer, we have hoped to encourage you to try it out as part of the ways in which you come to understand and learn from your practice. We also hope that trying some of the reflective exercises presented in the chapter has demonstrated the value of reflective writing in uncovering knowledge and your own approaches to practice that perhaps would not have surfaced in any other way. As professionals from all walks of health and social care practice move through their careers and build expertise and experiences that influence the way they work, there is a need to be able to recognize individual progress and development, and understand the ways in which we use ourselves in therapeutic contexts. As we become more advanced in our practice, it is usual for the power and responsibility for the working environment, for other practitioners, and for our clients and patients also to increase. As a result, the consequences of our decisions and actions may be more far-reaching and affect more people than earlier in our careers. The development of critical reflection as a way of working provides some safeguards for us in understanding the underpinning motivations and assumptions for our decisions and behaviour. Working as critical thinkers, and utilizing critical reflective writing strategies in a personal way, ensures that we are conscious of the rationale used for making decisions and for how we affect those we work with, whoever we may be. Critical reflective writing helps us to stay in touch with reality as a basis on which to build and ground our practice because it forces us to challenge our assumptions and explore alternatives to what may have become routine or customized practice. Finally, critical reflective writing helps us to validate ourselves as practitioners by recognizing our contribution to patient and client care through a window for exploring ourselves in a professional context.

Further reading

The past decade has seen the growth of reflective learning in programmes for pre-registration/qualification entry to the professional registers across the healthcare professions. The list below provides some examples reported in the literature.

- *Doctors*: Bethune and Brown (2007); Charon (2001); Grant et al. (2006); Rosenbaum, Ferguson and Broderick (2008).
- *Nurses*: Bowers and Jinks (2004); Harris (2008); Morgan, Rawlinson and Weaver (2006); Simpson and Courtney (2007).
- *Physiotherapists*: Sutton and Dalley (2008).
- *Radiographers*: Curtise, White and McKay (2008); Milinkovic and Field (2005).
- *Social workers*: Rai (2006); Swindell and Watson (2006); Taylor (2006); Waldman (2005).

Reflective moment

Now turn back to the aims that you identified at the start of the chapter. To what extent have they been met? Write a paragraph outlining the factual and practical knowledge you have acquired through reading this chapter and doing the exercises. Write a second paragraph identifying any aims which you feel were only partially met or not met at all. As in previous chapters, divide your page into three columns. Head the first column 'What I need to learn', and make a list of any outstanding issues which you would like to learn more about. For example, you might wish to find out more about the 'writing to learn' approach. Head the second column 'How I will learn it', and write down the ways in which your learning needs could be addressed; for example, through further reading, through attending study days, or through talking to other people. Head the third column 'How I will know that I have learnt it', and try to identify how you will know when you have met your needs.

5
Strategies for reflective writing

Melanie Jasper

Introduction

This chapter is about you, and how you can develop your writing within a critically reflective practice. Having looked at what reflective writing and writing critically may be in the last chapter, our aim here is to explore some writing strategies and techniques that might be employed to help you learn from, understand and develop your professional practice. Our aims for this chapter are therefore:

1. to explore various strategies for reflective writing as a means of critical reflection and of developing critical thinking;
2. to help you to explore ways of writing reflectively within your professional role, your personal development and to benefit client care; and
3. to help you plan to use reflective writing within research and your professional portfolio.

Reflective moment

Think carefully about our aims for Chapter 5. Now think about your own practice and how these aims might contribute towards developing it.

Based on our aims above, identify and write down some of your own, both in terms of what you hope to know and what you hope to be able to do after reading Chapter 5. We will return to these at the end of the chapter.

As this chapter is essentially about you, you will get the most out of it if you engage in the reflective activities as you go along. They are designed to help you build, incrementally, an understanding of yourself as a writer and how this knowledge can be used most effectively within your reflective writing related to your professional practice. You will find that there are many questions written into the text that follows, but few answers! These, by necessity, need to come from you.

Think about your own practice and how these aims might contribute towards developing it. For example, can you think of any ways that reflective writing may help you to explore a problem you have in practice? Think about your use of writing over the past few years – in what ways have you learnt about yourself and your practice as a result of this writing? Do you have to communicate through writing in your work? What would you like to do to make this more effective? Finally, do you have to keep a professional portfolio for any reason? Do you use reflective writing in any way within this?

It is important to remember that no single strategy will suit everyone, that there is no right and wrong to reflective writing, and that the adoption of a technique that is contrary to one's own personality, learning style and inclination is likely to be doomed to failure from the start. So, perhaps one way to start in identifying a writing strategy is to reflect on ways that we have written in the past.

Reflective moment

Have a look back at the answers you gave to the first reflective writing exercise in the previous chapter. In particular, think about what they say about the way that you usually go about writing.

Now make a list of all of the different types of writing that you can remember doing. This includes not only writing in an educational context, but writing for pleasure or for the purpose of communicating with others.

Which of these forms of writing did/do you enjoy, or get satisfaction out of the most? Try to write down the reasons why these are at the top of your list.

Now consider your approach to writing: What is your motivation for writing? Does it come from inside of you; are you intrinsically motivated, do you feel that you *have* to write for some reason that is driving you? Or are you extrinsically motivated; does the stimulus to write come from outside, maybe for reward, or for work, or for other people such as course work for lecturers?

Finding a writing strategy

Understanding how and why we write enables us to select ways of writing that may help us in reflecting. Sharples (1999) suggests that writers can be divided into 'discoverers' and 'planners' according to the two broad approaches that they take to their writing. Discoverers, he says, are:

> driven by engagement with the text. For them, self-understanding arises from writing. They may prefer to begin by scribbling out a draft that reveals their thoughts to them. Then, they often rework their text many times, reading and revising until it 'shapes up' to the constraints of the task and audience. The rhythm of their writing is often one of long periods of engaged composing, followed by extensive revision. (Sharples, 1999, p. 112)

In contrast, planners:

> are driven by reflection. For these people, writing flows from understanding. They spend a large proportion of their time on exploring ideas and on preparing mental or written plans. The plans guide composing and when there is a mismatch they either edit the text or revise the plan. Their rhythm of composing is, typically, one of rapid alternation between engagement and reflection, continually making minor adjustments to keep plan and text in harmony. (Sharples, 1999, p. 113)

It is, of course, rare that we would all fall neatly into one category or the other. However, you may recognize some of the characteristics that you listed in the last reflective writing exercise from these descriptions. How will this help with our own writing? By recognizing the ways in which we have approached writing in the past, we may be able to anticipate ways in which we can make writing work for us; equally, we may be able to evaluate particular ways of approaching writing and make a reasoned decision that they are not for us. This is very important in being comfortable with your writing, in choosing to write rather than being compelled to write because you are expected to. By understanding your own relationship with writing, you are more likely to view it as a positive way of learning, rather than as something that is imposed upon you by an outside force.

Sharples (1999) goes further in his identification of writing styles by citing a study by Wyllie (1993) which looked at student and academic writers and attempted to classify them by the strategies they

Table 5.1 Features of different strategies for writing

Writing characteristics	Watercolourist	Architect	Bricklayer	Sketcher	Oil painter
Overall type of writer Strategy for writing	Planner Single draft of whole paper with minimal revision, usually sequential	Planner (external) Plan mostly before writing, then write, then review	Planner/discoverer Polish one sentence, paragraph or section before moving to the next	Discoverer/planner Rough plan, revise later	Discoverer Jot down ideas as they occur, organise later, rarely sequential
Strategy for planning	Plan in head with broad headings	Detailed plan. Compose with broad headings	Type of planning depends on combination of strategies	Compose with broad headings	Compose with broad headings. Sometimes have a rough plan
Order of writing	Always sequential	Often sequential	Sometimes sequential	Sometimes sequential, sometimes jump about	Sometimes sequential, sometimes jump about
Starting writing	Rarely start easiest part first	Sometimes start easiest part first	Rarely start easiest part first	Occasionally start the easiest part first	Often start easiest part first
Revision strategy	Little revision - some changes	Revise a fair amount, mainly at sentence level	Fair amount of revision, mainly spelling, grammar and re-sequencing	Much revision, mainly meaning and sequence changes, and sentence level	Much revision, particularly meaning and sentence
Correction strategy	Tend not to correct	Rarely correct as they go, mainly on printout	Correct at both stages, but mainly later	Correct as they go, also later	Correct as they go, but mainly later
Strategy for reviewing work	Tend to review more on screen than other strategies	Tend to review on printout	Will review on screen, but prefer printout	Review on screen and on printout	Least tendency to review on screen, mainly printout
Relationship with screen	Don't find screen restrictive. Rarely lose overall sense of the text	Occasionally find screen too restrictive	Often find screen restrictive. Often lose overall sense of the text	Occasionally find screen restrictive	Occasionally find screen restrictive

Source: Adapted from Sharples (1999, pp. 116–17), from original work by Wyllie (1993).

used as writers. Table 5.1 illustrates what we all really know at heart: that different people approach writing in different ways. Sometimes, however, we need reminding of this, such as when others appear to effortlessly sit at a word processor, or with pen and paper in front of them, and write thousands of words, while the rest of us are making just one more cup of coffee, or putting another load of washing on the line just to put off the moment when we have to sit down in front of an empty screen and do something with it! The different strategies that Wyllie (1993) identified may help us to understand more about the creative processes that we use in writing, and to accept that we can all be equally successful in writing provided that we find a method that suits us, rather than attempting to conform to one that someone else imposes.

Reflective moment

In the last chapter we asked you to consider your previous experiences of writing, why you have written in the past, and what your attitude to writing has been, and is now. The reasons for doing this will be, we hope, becoming clear to you.

What we would like you to do now is to focus on the types of writing that you have enjoyed in the past – those where you have gained some sort of pleasure or satisfaction, or where you can say that you have gained something from the experience of writing, even though the actual act of doing it may have been difficult for you.

Now recall those previous experiences, write down the features that made them rewarding, and use them to plan some writing strategies that you could use in the future.

Understanding the reasons why you have enjoyed writing is important because you can plan to write reflectively in a style that suits you and with which you feel comfortable. For example, if you like a definite structure to your writing you may like to utilize one or more of the reflective frameworks outlined in this book (see Chapter 3), such as those suggested by Sarah Stephenson (Holm and Stephenson, 1994) or Graham Gibbs (1988). This brings us back to whether you fall into the category of being a discoverer or a planner. For many people, the idea of writing to a predetermined structure is what puts them off writing, because they find it difficult to reduce their experiences into categories. For them, the types of writing that fall into the 'creative' category are more likely to engage them. Similarly, you will find that one single strategy is not appropriate for all the times that you want to write, and it is useful to consider trying other ways of writing that appear to be better suited to whatever it is that you are writing about, or the outcomes you want to achieve from the writing.

It is important, however, to remember the reflective component as being a key issue here; that we are reflecting in order to learn and to enable us to take a different perspective. This is hard work, since we are deliberately deciding to explore our own reality and our own experiences, and at times this may be painful or reveal things to us that have been hidden. Equally, there can be great joy in writing, such as in unlocking secrets that have puzzled us for some time, or when we learn things about ourselves and those around us that we like and can celebrate. Some excellent examples of the ways in which written reflection can help practitioners to make sense of events from their past are explored in Bolton's (2006) book looking at writing for personal development.

Finding something to write about

Initially, finding a subject for writing can be one of the hardest hurdles to overcome. In terms of reflective writing, we need to find a stimulus to write and to write about something that will enable us to learn. One of the terms for that 'something' is a *critical incident*. To some extent, this is an unfortunate term for those engaged in healthcare, because the word 'critical' has particular associations with life-threatening crises or dramatic events. However, if we see critical as meaning 'important' or something that has significance for us in some way and stands out in our memory, we can start to refocus what we see as a *critical* incident. Similarly, for an event or an occurrence to be seen as an incident, we would logically have to be able to describe it; it would need to be an event that had boundaries that we could define, and certain actions or activities that went on within it that could be encapsulated. Many of the structured strategies for reflection that you will meet in this book are based on the concept of the critical incident. The classic definition of a critical incident was phrased by John Flanagan:

> By an incident is meant any observable human activity that is sufficiently complete in itself to permit inferences and predictions to be made about the person performing the act. To be critical, an incident must

occur in a situation where the purpose or intent of the act seems fairly clear to the observer and where its consequences are sufficiently definite to leave little doubt concerning its effects. (Flanagan, 1954, p. 327)

This definition is useful in enabling us to identify episodes that fulfil these criteria so that a concrete description can be written and explored reflectively.

This suggests, however, that critical incidents need to be relatively small or minor occurrences. For many of us who write reflectively, the topics of our writing are wider than single definable incidences, such as relationships with our clients or colleagues, the whole of the history of dealing with one particular patient, designing a curriculum, or a complete experience at work; the list is endless. To some extent these can be regarded as critical incidents because, for whatever reason, they can be seen to fulfil the first set of criteria in Flanagan's definition. However, they do not readily comply with the criteria in the second sentence, which imply that there are easily definable and finite consequences or actions. Many of the reflective writing strategies used within education use critical incidents, and this is where many practitioners will experience reflective writing for the first time. It is undoubtedly an extremely useful technique when used to identify and explore experiences that can be described in Flanagan's way, but limiting ourselves to critical incidents may narrow the reflective focus for our writing.

A second way of identifying the subject of our writing can be found in Atkins and Murphy's (1994) work, which suggests that there are three stages to the reflective process (summarized in Table 5.2).

The first of these is where the stimulus for reflection occurs, and is identified as:

An awareness of uncomfortable feelings or thoughts. This arises from a realisation that, in a situation, the knowledge one was applying was not sufficient in itself to explain what was happening in that unique situation. (Atkins and Murphy, 1994, p. 1189).

Table 5.2 Summary of Atkins and Murphy's (1994) stages of the reflective process

Stage	Description
1	An awareness of uncomfortable feelings and thoughts
2	A critical analysis of the situation, which is constructive and involves an examination of feelings and knowledge
3	Development of a new perspective on the situation

While, undoubtedly, much reflection is stimulated by unpleasant or uncomfortable feelings, this one sentence has pervaded the notion of reflection in nursing in particular to such an extent as to provide a negative connotation to the whole process. Many practitioners have been introduced to the reflective process through the idea that reflective practice arises solely from things that have caused discomfort. Of course, nothing can be further from the truth! We tend to build on success, and in the past many of us unconsciously repeated actions and ways of working that had been previously successful, and avoided ones that had not. The overt use of reflective processes, and of critical reflection as a whole, is to enable us to learn deliberatively from our experiences and to enable us to identify action that can be taken in the future.

Thus, reflective writing does not need to be restricted to identifying critical incidents that have caused us to feel uncomfortable. Rather, reflection is concerned with anything that happens to us that *we want to write about for some reason*. It is not necessarily the subject that is the key here; it is the fact that we want to write about it! Hence, it may be very useful to commit problems to paper, particularly those that tend to get stuck in our head and which we go over and over in a seemingly unrelenting spiral. However, these are by no means the majority of our experiences, and in fact most of our time is spent in positive activities that are very successful.

So, to return to the question that we started this section with: what do we write about? The simple answer is that we can write about anything that has happened to us. Perhaps a more pertinent question, however, is how do we select from those experiences so that we are not attempting to catalogue the whole of our day? For us, the key to answering this question concerns the significance of the experience within our daily lives. If something is important to you, for whatever reason, then it is worth writing about. In fact, it is likely that you will *want* to write about it! Taking this approach frees us from the rules imposed by others on our writing. We learn to write for ourselves, and in so doing, we *use* writing as a means of self-discovery.

Reflective moment

Close your eyes and think back to yesterday. Briefly scan in your mind the whole day and review all of the things that happened to you. Now, write down the 10 things that stand out as the most important to you.

Why did you write these things down as opposed to all of the other things that happened to you? What is significant about these 10 that separated them out from the other things that you did?

Look at your list more closely. Have you imposed some sort of value system on these experiences that isolates the activity from the experience of it? For instance, did you write 'I went to work' because it has social and economic significance, or did you write about an experience at work that had emotional significance?

Look back at your list again, and think about it with a different focus. This time, think about the emotional content of the experiences, and delete any that do not involve some sort of feelings about them. Now replace these with the equivalent number of experiences. For instance, you may replace 'Went to work' with 'I bought an ice-cream and sat for five minutes in the sunshine relaxing to eat it.'

Now you have a different list, and one that probably has a special significance for you as a person, rather than you as an individual playing a combination of different roles that impose sets of rules on you. Take each one of these experiences separately and try to write down why they are significant for you, what the emotional component of them is, and what you have learnt about yourself as a result of them.

Of course, it is unlikely that we would be able to write in this way every day, but if writing becomes a way of life, it can be a habitual technique for exploring, experiencing and valuing our world. What we do need to be able to do, though, is to shed many of the externally imposed rules and regulations that we have learnt about writing as a result of our past experiences, and view writing for ourselves as value-free (unless we choose to impose values) yet valuable to us; to use styles and strategies for writing that are comfortable for us and suit the need for which we are writing. Reflective writing can be in any style that we want it to be, unless we are writing for other people who have defined a style for us. In the next section we briefly look at different styles and strategies for writing, all of which can be used for writing reflectively if the other stages of the reflective cycle are superimposed on them.

An easy way of doing this is to use the 'three-a-day' technique. Simply ask yourself 'What are the three most successful/most enjoyable/most exciting/least successful, etc, things that I did today?' Try not to intellectualize, but just let things come into your head, as your sub-conscious is doing the work of shifting experiences into a hierarchy of importance for you. Then select one of these as the focus for your reflective activity. With practice, this becomes an habitual activity, and one that you can do at any time to help you think about what experiences require your attention and warrant further exploration through critical reflection and reflective writing.

Styles and strategies for reflective writing

We have all received the less than helpful advice that the best way to start writing is to simply sit down and do it! Unfortunately, as a strategy, this is probably correct, but there are ways of doing it that are less threatening than simply being faced with a blank screen or piece of paper. Our intentions in the previous sections were to help you understand the processes of writing and come to an awareness of previous writing experiences so they can be used to facilitate writing in the future. We cannot reiterate too many times that there is no one right way of writing; the only correct way is the way that works for you. However, the styles and types of writing that follow may help to get you thinking about some possible strategies that you can utilize.

Analytical and critical strategies

We have called these analytical strategies because the process of analysis and synthesis is integral to the process of writing. These strategies have in common the notion of attempting to stand back from an event while acknowledging the personal and emotional commitment. The style of writing alternates between description, recognition of the features of the event, analysis, exploration and synthesis. Analytical strategies are characterized by dialogue, or having a conversation with oneself in which argument and counterpoint are proposed and written. It is the development of the subjective reality of an experience that moves its exploration from being solely analytical (i.e., in relation to the belief in an objective reality) to being critically reflective, or as Johns (2000, p. 34) expressed it:

a window through which the practitioner can view and focus the self within the context of her own lived experience in ways that enable her to confront, understand and work towards resolving the contradictions within her practice and between what is desirable and actual practice.

Journal writing

Keeping a journal is perhaps the commonest analytical strategy to be found in the professional and educational literature and is probably the easiest place to start writing, in that a journal kept specifically for one's own personal and private use overcomes all of the barriers about judgement and other people having access to our writing.

The term 'journal', as used here, refers to writing about, and exploring experiences in practice on an incremental basis. It is analytical, and often critical in nature, and thus differs from diaries or logs in that they tend to be descriptive in recording events that have happened but not necessarily explorative in nature. Cunliffe (2004) suggests that journaling is a powerful way to engage people in their own learning and for surfacing tacit knowledge from practice. Others suggest that reflective writing is an enabling strategy that improves analytical and critical thinking; builds self-awareness; surfaces, articulates and helps us to rethink our conceptualizations of the world; and enables connectivity between previously disparate sets of information (Locke and Brazelton, 1997; Jasper, 1999). It is the processes engaged in when writing in this way that enable these developments and understandings and contribute to the practitioner's personal and professional development and identity; moreover, the end result is likely to be improved patient outcomes (Jasper, 1999; Shapiro, Kasman and Shafer, 2006).

When experimenting with journal writing it is worth bearing in mind the processes and features of writing that we discussed earlier. Remember, it is vital that you are comfortable with the processes and strategies that you adopt for your own reflective writing, and that you make the decisions about how and what you write. This does not, of course, mean that the analytical and critical processes, or the insights developed and conclusions reached will lack challenge, or indeed be comfortable! Think of the difference between being confident and competent in a technical procedure, and the reality of doing it in practice. The latter may well throw up individual differences and challenges that ask you to draw on other knowledge, skill and experience as a consequence, despite your own tacit understanding of the procedure in the first place.

In terms of structures, there are of course no rules, but there are a few things to think about to ensure that you plan to be successful in your journal writing rather than it becoming a bit like the majority of New Year's resolutions. First of all, think about the practicalities of where and when, you are likely to write. Does this means that your journal needs to be portable? Will you use a notebook to write in, loose-leaf paper pads, or a computer? If the latter, will it be handheld, a laptop or fixed in place?

Second, can you use the features of writing we have already discussed as a mental checklist, or even as a physical design to enable you to structure your writing as you progress?

Third, will you want to use a model or framework to structure your writing and hence your analytical activity, or would you prefer to be more responsive to the issues as they arise and use a reflective framework such as those suggested in Chapter 3? Or perhaps, you may have the confidence to develop your own style of reflective writing which enables you to explore different perspectives of an experience according to the purpose of your writing.

As reflective activity however, it is worth attempting to incorporate physical structures into the journal that allow you to return to the entry, re-read and annotate it with further thoughts. One way of doing this is advocated by Holly (1984), who suggests that a new page is started for each entry, with the description of the incident written on the left-hand page, and the right-hand page being used for the reflective analysis and writing on later occasions. This enables the writer to return and add further entries to develop the reflection. The journal then becomes a dialogue with ourselves as we return to it, up-date and add to it as a record of our work. Journals rarely contain the physical evidence to support the learning being identified, and indeed this is not the primary function of the journal. Rather, the journal is intended to provide a medium for the writer to have a personal conversation where issues can be explored within the safety of personal boundaries.

Many sorts of journal entries could form the basis of your professional portfolio or evidence of continuing professional development required by all the professional bodies for periodic re-registration. It would clearly demonstrate your on-going professional development and competence and provide evidence of accountable and ethical practice. This is particularly so if you want to show how you have learnt from an experience and changed your practice in some way, or, for instance, if you attended a study day and have incorporated learning from that event into how you practice.

Reflective reviews and critical incident analyses

In contrast to journal writing, reflective reviews and critical incident analyses are where most of us will have had our first experiences of writing reflectively from course requirements within formal professional education. As a result, this will have been many practitioners' only experience, and may have coloured their views about the usefulness of the techniques in relation to their own continuing professional development outside the formal setting. Writing in this way when you are required to do it, with the parameters set by others and over which you have no control, limits its usefulness as a strategy. However, once freed from boundaries imposed by others, the techniques of exploring a particular experience in detail enables a wealth of understanding to develop through being in control of the process.

Many writers choose to build up a series of case studies using reflective reviews or critical incident technique. This is often combined with a strategy for reflection that breaks the incident and the reflective cycle down into separate sections and uses key prompts to direct the analysis. This is useful for the beginning writer especially, as it provides a framework of specific questions, whether from a named model or created by the writer before they start writing, to address a particular, pre-identified aspect of the problem. For instance, you might be attempting to explore why you took the particular decisions that you did, or you might want to explore your emotional response to an incident. You may want to relive a situation to see whether you could have handled it differently or have caused a different outcome. Or you may want to find out why something went so spectacularly well that you want to be able to repeat it. This can provide you with the starting point for constructing your own list of questions that you want answered through your reflective exploration. It also has the added advantage of freeing the writer from creating their own analytical strategies, but can be inhibiting for those who do not think in the way asked of them by the predetermined structure. The key to using critical incident analysis is that the reflective cycle is completed in terms of defining strategies for action or reflecting on the new insight that has taken place.

A wealth of understanding can occur from deliberately exploring the same experience or case study from different perspectives. For instance you could explore:

- the evidence base/knowledge used to inform your practical decision-making;
- the learning and teaching strategies used with a student to enable their skills and understanding of the incident to develop;
- your role in the multidisciplinary team in managing the client's care;

- the outcome(s) of the course(s) of action taken;
- your emotional responses to the incident and the consequences of these;
- implications of an incident for your practice, personal and professional development; and
- your own learning from the incident

And those are just for starters!

Dialogical writing

This is a form of writing where the writer consciously sets out to have a conversation with themselves, proposing ideas and counter-ideas in a series of questions and answers, or through graded discussion that is moved forward through the writing. The questions themselves arise from the writing, rather than from a pre-determined framework, freeing the writer to explore an incident in a more free-form way, and to go wherever the mind goes in response to what has already been written. This means that issues raised will be followed up, with such questions as 'why did I do that?' or 'what else could I have done?' or 'what am I going to do with the knowledge that I have gained from exploring this incident?' This strategy avoids the security of the pre-written frameworks, which have the danger of enabling the reflector to move on to the next set of questions without fully going with their instinct and listening to themselves and what their writing is saying to them.

Making a case

Although similar to dialogical writing, the purpose of this is to create an argument that will persuade another person of the value of the viewpoint. This, in many ways, is very close to an academic writing style. This technique is particularly useful in enabling a writer to see another person's point of view, or in reinforcing the features of a case to present a particular viewpoint as the result of a reasoned exploration of evidence and knowledge, or even an ethical or philosophical position. This taps into the notion of critical reflection extremely well, as it picks up on the notion of the social construction of reality, as opposed to the idea that there is an objective reality. There are always several different interpretations of incidents and experiences – deliberately attempting to argue a case opposite to the one we would naturally choose, as in a debate, is an excellent exercise in critical thinking and developing perspectives.

Creative strategies

These techniques separate out the descriptive, personal and emotional components from the analytical and reflective. They are classed as creative because they involve using the imagination and transforming experience away from the rational ways of analysis that character-ize the above group, and move the writer into imagination and meta-phor as a way of creating insight and facilitating learning. Often, the artefact produced is not a descriptive account, but may be a reworked account of the experience that is used separately for reflection and analysis after its creation. These techniques are particularly useful for enabling practitioners to deal with difficult and emotive situations that need the emotional response to be resolved before they can move on to exploring the issue more analytically and critically.

Writing the unsent letter or email

Have you ever written a letter or email and then never sent it? An unsent letter can perform some very useful functions in enabling us to write in a style that is far-removed from the analytical styles of the previous strategies, and provides us with a way of capturing emo-tions and feelings in their rawest forms. Unsent letters are often used where experiences have been particularly painful, and in order for the writer to explore them, she needs first to draw on the cathartic effect of pouring emotions onto paper. The unsent letter technique seems to be very effective when the imagined recipient of the letter is the per-son who has caused the problem; for instance, an incident with a col-league or manager, a difficult client, or a teacher who appears to have been unreasonable. What is unlikely to be recorded in this technique is a description of the event in any linear form, if it is there at all. Nor is it likely that the whole event will be conveyed to the reader.

The advantage of this technique is that the writer can literally write exactly what she thinks to the imagined recipient of the let-ter, yet there is safety in the knowledge that it will not be sent. At times, we have experiences that are so painful emotionally that we are not able to explore them rationally close to the time that they occur. Using the unsent letter to record feelings and emotions can be a way of taking the first step of creating some sort of permanent record of the event, which will stimulate memories when it is re-read at a later date. However, it may also have the effect of enabling the writer to start to deal with those emotions simply through the process of writing them down on paper.

There is one note of caution here however, for those people who routinely use email as a form of communication. It is all too easy to be provoked into writing an emotional, and often unwise message to an antagonist, and using it to vent your feelings in very graphic ways. It is also very easy to press the 'send' button, before really considering the consequences of that action. While the unsent letter requires a lot more effort to put in the post, the unsent email is extremely easy to send. Emails are permanent records (even when deleted!) and may be used in disputes between colleagues and employers. Even if not used in formal procedures, accusatory and inflammatory emails cause tension and ill-feeling and are considered to be a form of bullying. They can also destroy relationships and trust between people, when sorting out the same issue face-to-face would have resolved it and maintained the status quo. The golden rule with email is to not write anything to anybody that you would not want used as evidence against you in a grievance, employment tribunal or court case! The other golden rule is to take time out following an emotional incident before writing an email response. If you have to write immediately, delete before sending, or save as a draft and re-read after a good night's sleep!

Writing to another person

This is really a variation on the above strategy, but instead of imagining writing to the person involved in the event, the writer writes as if telling another person with whom she is familiar, be it a friend, a relative or even a respected teacher. This technique enables the writer to put her own point of view, but this tends to be modified by the imagined effect or authority of the recipient. It is more likely that this type of letter will include a description of what has happened, or it may include ideas and propositions from the writer that take a dialogue forward. Again, this sort of exercise tricks our subconscious into providing a different perspective on an incident, as, depending on the person whom we picture writing to, we may start to question our motives or change elements of the story to present a different picture. We will also tend to edit the story in some way, maybe to show us in a more flattering light, or to justify our perspective, and yet that action alone will start us questioning our behaviours and exploring them more critically.

Writing as the other

With this technique, the writer attempts to put herself in the place of the other person in the event, and tell the story from her point of view. This can be useful in attempting to get a person to move beyond barriers that are preventing her from analyzing a situation, particularly if the writing is facilitated by using key questions. This can be supplemented by the writer writing about the event first from her own viewpoint, and then from that of another, or even from all of the players in the interaction.

This technique identifies an issue within the proponents of reflective practice as to whether it is possible to reflect upon someone's actions and emotions. As a subjective practice, critical reflection surfaces assumptions and encourages reconceptualization of events from the knowledge and experience of the person writing it. That person can only understand another person's viewpoint from the way they experience the expression of it, or their own subjective experience, and cannot ever be sure that their interpretation is what the other person's is or was. Assuming motivation, or causality, and making value judgments about the other's perceived view must be done with the clear knowledge that they may be wrong. Therefore, many advocates of reflective writing caution against attempting to see events through another person's eyes, in recognition that this imagined view may become another version of reality that did not ever exist for anybody. However, while it is impossible to 'get inside someone else's head', the activity of attempting to see an event from a different point of view often enables insight to develop.

Storytelling

In this technique, the writer writes as if creating a story for an audience, either to be read aloud or to be read silently. In this way, the unconscious thoughts that we were not aware of at the time of an experience can be brought to the fore and acknowledged. Metaphor can be used to recreate the experience, where the writer is able to impose her perspective on the account. Examples of this strategy may include giving the key players fictional names that reflect how the writer sees them, or imputing motive onto players where the writer cannot have had access to this.

In many ways, all forms of reflective writing can be seen as storytelling, as we re-create and articulate the incident from a particular perspective. Thus, every version tells a different 'story'. In fact, valuable insights can be achieved if several people involved in an incident all write it from their own perspective, and these are then considered alongside each other.

Charon (2001), and Alcauskas and Charon (2008) talk, in particular from working with medical students, about reflective writing as a way of developing narrative competence in doctors. They suggest that 'reflective writers study their own decision-making, feelings, behaviours, interactions, and gaps in knowledge and skill. Reflecting on one's own practice coincides with the development of insight into one's own educational needs and the ability to better practice well autonomously' (Alcauskas and Charon, 2008). Other professions traditionally located in the 'hard science' educational paradigm, such as physiotherapy and radiography, are moving to incorporate narrative techniques into the preparation of practitioners to develop more holistic approaches to practice and their interactions with clients. For instance, Brady, Corbie-Smith and Branch (2002) state that 'narratives provided us with an understanding of the interplay among residents' interactions with patients, their own personal issues, and their struggles during several discrete stages of their professional development'.

Both Bolton (2006) and Shapiro, Kasman and Shafer (2006) use a technique of working with groups of practitioners, often from multidisciplinary origins, through a two-stage process of individual writing followed by group discussion and public exploration of the narrative story. Shapiro, Kasman and Shafer (2006) have identified this as the writing/reading/listening process which results in individual development through vulnerability and risk-taking, mindfulness and witnessing leading to personal self-awareness and growth. Bolton (2006) names her approach as 'through the looking glass', suggesting this self-awareness develops as a result of 'seeing' different views of oneself through others' eyes. These techniques explicitly move from the private nature of reflective writing into the public forum, where group challenge and differing perspective can help the writer move on from an individualized analysis and conclusions regarding an event or experience. These approaches also help the development of critical reflection, in that others asking questions will help the writer to think in alternative ways and consider the assumptions on which their decisions and conclusions were based.

Poetry as reflective writing

Poetry is perhaps the archetypal style of creative writing, where the features of writing reflectively as having meaning for ourselves are most acutely obvious.

All of these techniques are aimed at enabling the individual to learn through reflective writing and other related reflective activity in order to develop critical reflective skills related to practice. However, reflective writing can also be used collectively by a number of people to develop teams and alternative approaches to problem-solving.

Writing reflectively with others

Most of the writing we do is as individuals, writing of, from or about ourselves. We are all familiar with written artifacts that have several contributors, such as a newspaper, or a set of patient records. These are built up from individual contributions, and the sum total of these tells a story that is more than any one of the writers may have known. As a result of more than one person writing from their own perspective, the subject of their writing becomes rounder and fuller.

Think of the possibilities of this approach for reflective writing. We already see jointly authored papers and books (and indeed this book is such an example, where three people have contributed from their own expertise and experience and produced a final product that includes much more than any one of us could have envisaged); but the techniques and models of reflective writing can also be used by people working together to explore phenomena or incidents in many ways, and with varying outcomes. Indeed, Orland-Barak (2005) suggests that collaborative writing leads to higher levels of reflectivity as a result of the group thinking and discussion processes which results in what she identifies as 'discussions of the untold'.

Any of the frameworks of reflection explored and presented throughout the book are just as suitable for joint writing as for use by an individual. For instance, Kim's (1999) framework could be used by two people to explore an incident that happened to both of them, and may help to resolve any difficulties between them as a result. The writing aspect of it is important in that equal weight would be given to both people's 'stories' so that a full picture would emerge. Similarly, a joint record could be made of a supervisory relationship, with both supervisor and supervisee contributing to the same document from their own perspectives. Many authors provide examples of dialogical writing used between supervisor or mentor and student to ensure effective learning in practice. Harris (2008) suggests 'scaffolding' deep learning through reflective writing between student and tutor. Plack and Greenberg (2005) suggest that the role of the supervisor is to pose questions and challenge the student/writer as guidance for further development and to avoid journals becoming descriptive diaries. These techniques for collaborative writing would provide all of the advantages of writing over discussion, and indeed can be used for supervision at a distance.

Reflective writing can also be used incrementally with a group of people who work within a team, or who come together for a specific purpose. Imagine, for instance, the painstaking work that is done by a ward team looking after a long-term patient. In addition to the records used in documenting care, the team could create a living book for that patient in which views are recorded on treatments and approaches to care, breakthroughs described, new paths taken, and so on. DeMarco et al. (2005) used group writing as a way of working through and decreasing negative workplace behaviours; while Alterio (2004) provides evidence of the development of practice-related learning and personal philosophies arising from the group processes operating in the public arena, providing multiple perspectives on situations and events. In this way, practice knowledge is documented as it is created, with evidence and records of alternatives and issues as they arise. A similar approach can be taken for new initiatives or changes in an environment, particularly where it is difficult for all members of the team to get together to explore the issues between them. In this way, views can be built up through an ongoing dialogue, with all members having the opportunity to put their point of view and have it acknowledged.

These are only a few suggestions for the ways in which reflective writing can be used in the public domain between two or more people. Many others that can add richness to writing reflectively are possible, which could contribute towards the creation of knowledge from experience.

Reflective moment

Are there any issues in your work environment that you feel would be suitable for a collaborative reflective writing approach? Discuss with your colleagues how issues that appear to be stagnant could be moved forward by providing a book for people to record their ideas and thoughts in, and to record progress made.

Further reading

All of these techniques are developed further elsewhere. Chris Johns' (2000) work typifies journal writing, and is particularly useful for providing guides for structured reflection. Johns has, more recently, moved into an auto-ethnographic approach through narrative and performance. Similarly, Ira Progoff (1975) and Mary Holly (1984) have made useful contributions to strategies for reflective writing in journals.

Reflective writing in professional portfolios

All registrants with the Health Professions Council, the General Social Care Council and the Nursing and Midwifery Council are now required to maintain a professional portfolio in order to demonstrate evidence of their regular updating and professional development. Post-qualifying medical education and training is also increasingly expecting the development of reflective understanding demonstrated in written reflective approaches within documentation and assessment (Grant et al., 2006; Rosenbaum, Ferguson and Muir Gray, (2008). There is an expectation from the professional bodies that reflective writing will be utilized to explore learning experiences and to show how they are informing and being incorporated into practice. An essential and critical difference between a portfolio *per se* and the strategies of reflective writing, is that a portfolio is designed and constructed to portray a picture of its creator and, as such, is likely to be open to public scrutiny in some form. While reflective writing may well be included in, and form an essential part of, a portfolio, it is the responsibility of the writer to make clear decisions as to what part of the portfolio is selected for others to read.

Portfolios are usually created for a specific purpose, such as course work, as a record of practice, and so on. As such, specific criteria are published as to what the portfolio should contain. It is usual that the content needs to provide evidence of the owner of the portfolio meeting the stated criteria. In educational portfolios, these will usually be phrased as learning outcomes or core constituents such as attendance certificates, job descriptions or records of work completed. Guidance and guidelines for portfolios created for specific purposes will clearly originate from those bodies requiring them to be created, and are thus outside the brief of this book. What we would like to explore further here is the way that reflective writing can be used within a portfolio to provide evidence of learning and development of the person in relation to their professional role.

We have seen from the previous chapters that much of the literature on reflection, reflective practice and ideas about knowledge arising from practice is located in the world of education. Authors in the professional and academic press report on reflective strategies used with students, and there is also a plethora of individual accounts of reflective writing in practice. These often make the connection between theories of reflection and real-life examples, but little attention has been paid to the processes of reflective writing within the reflective cycle, or to how practitioners use writing within their own practice when it is not required of them as part of a course. It seems to be assumed that writing will occur, but scant attention is paid to how to do it, or to how practitioners are actually doing it when they are not monitored or facilitated in some way.

Think about your own portfolio (assuming that you have one – if you haven't you may like to use these questions to think about how you might construct one).

- Why do you keep a portfolio?
- What have you got in it?
- How have you structured it?
- Why have you structured it in this way?
- How do you use reflective writing in your portfolio?
- How do you use the learning achieved within your practice?

In the sections above we have deliberately focused on the micro-strategies that can be used for reflective writing, without assuming that they are being used within any particular framework or model for reflective activity. To us, it is crucial that frameworks and models are used as tools to guide and help, rather than as prescriptive and standardized check lists of questions used for every occasion. Being critically reflective means, at the very beginning, being able to consider alternatives and make conscious selections of courses of action as appropriate to need rather than following a pre-set plan simply because it exists. The same goes for selecting a framework to use for reflecting – the same criteria need to apply to selecting this tool for practice as for any other clinical decision you make. If your tendency is to always use the same framework to structure your reflective activity, now is a good time to explore why this is and think about being more inclusive!

Within portfolios, the use of frameworks or models can play the same role as when you are using reflection in any other context. They will help you through the processes of reflection by asking specific questions in a set order. It is therefore important to select the framework that will enable you to achieve the purpose of your reflective activity. When choosing a reflective framework or model to write through, it may be helpful to ask yourself the following questions:

- What is the focus of this particular reflective activity? For example, an event or experience, a problem or challenge that already exists, an anticipated future challenge;
- What am I trying to achieve, what outcome am I expecting? For example, personal or professional learning, ideas for changing practice or practice development, alternative courses of action; and
- What sorts of questions do I need to be asked to get me to this outcome? For example, do these need to explore your emotional reactions, your knowledge base, your beliefs and values, your assumptions.

These three questions should help you to consider selecting from the range of frameworks available, or spur you on to create your own set of questions that will get you to your expected end point.

The process of writing through these as a portfolio entry will serve several purposes. First, you will have worked your way reflectively through an issue that has been challenging you in some way. Second, you will have created a reasoned discussion of how you arrived at the conclusions you reached over the issue. This can be used to demonstrate your accountability as a professional practitioner and show how you base your practice in the best available evidence and experiential learning. Third, you will have a permanent record of how you practice reflectively, which may, or may not also incorporate some forms of evidence that you actually have achieved what you say you have achieved. This latter point is particularly important when you are writing portfolios for assessment purposes and need to prove that you have achieved certain learning outcomes or reached standards of competence within your practice.

The issue of the collection, and amount, of evidence that is included in a portfolio is often a difficult one to resolve. Of course, many portfolio entries will not require any evidence at all – after all, your portfolio might well be simply a private collection of your writings, created for your own purposes and used to that effect. However, most professional practitioners registered with a regulatory body will need to compile some sort of a portfolio against which they can be measured as fulfilling continuing professional development and competence requirements. Hence, it is important to consider the ways that evidence can be incorporated within the portfolio without it taking over and the portfolio looking like a mobile filing cabinet!

Perhaps the simplest way of looking at evidence is to consider it as 'proving' something about you. So, if you are claiming that you attended a study day, the evidence will be the certificate of attendance. However, this is not sufficient to be able to claim that you have *learnt* from attending that day in order to be able to count this as professional development, so you need to link that attendance to how you have used the knowledge or skill arising within your practice. The most obvious way of doing this would be to write reflectively following the study day on what new knowledge you have gained, how this supplements or challenges your existing knowledge, and how you plan to incorporate this into your practice. This may mean making changes to procedures or techniques that you use; it may mean reviewing standardized protocols in the light of new evidence; it may mean training others in new techniques – the list is probably endless. This gives you a prescription for action as a result of the initial reflective writing. Next, the action needs to be carried through and then evaluated, with further journal or portfolio entries documenting the progress being made. In this way, you use your portfolio dynamically to work through successive action research and change cycles that provide evidence not only of your part in the practice change, but which also records your own learning and development as a practitioner. Thus, you are creating the evidence as you progress through the process. You may even supplement this with testimonials from your manager, team or colleagues, clients and their families, or even by creating spin-off entries in the portfolio. For instance, you may choose to write up a case study of one particular client that you work with; or perhaps document differences that changes to practice have made on the environment in which you work.

Although there is no simple answer to the question of how much evidence to include in a portfolio, it needs to be sufficient to prove that what you are claiming is indeed true to an outside observer. That person may be a colleague, your manager, a teacher or even the professional body. The acid test though, is to show how the evidence is linked to the reflective activity that makes the case that you are presenting. Evidence will not talk by itself. Evidence can be interpreted in a multitude of ways – just think how two clever barristers can interpret the same evidence to support both prosecution and defence cases in a court case – so it is up to you, as the writer, to ensure that the evidence you select to use creates the picture of you that you want to present.

Writing reflectively within a portfolio needs to serve the purpose in your working life that you want it to serve. Like most reflective writing, it is not a strategy that can be imposed on a practitioner – the person needs to embrace the processes of reflective writing as central to the way they practice, and to incorporate it as one of the tools they use in their everyday working life.

Further reading

Jasper (2006) contains chapters on reflective writing and building professional portfolios that will provide practical advice, techniques and strategies beyond what has been included in this chapter.

Reflective moment

This chapter has deliberately focussed on the practical techniques and strategies that can be adopted within reflective writing. Being critical in this writing process involves being willing to explore different ways of doing things in order to find out different things. If you do things in the same way every time, you will end up with the same outcome, resulting in boredom and stagnation. Take a look back over the strategies and techniques suggested in this chapter and make a list of them. Quickly rank them on a scale of one to ten, first on how interesting and attractive they are to you, and second on how likely you are to use each of them. Now, revisit those judgements and ask yourself why you responded in the ways you have. Is there something to do with familiarity and working in a comfort zone that influenced your decisions? Do you need to make a decision to try something new?

Conclusion

We hope that this chapter has enabled you to develop your understanding of how different ways and approaches to writing can be used to create differing understandings and perspectives on your experience to precipitate action and change in your practice. One of the challenges for us as teachers and facilitators over the past decade has been in finding ways of helping our students and the practitioners with whom we work to understand and develop the capacity to lift their reflective activity to a level which could be recognized as 'critical'. These are skills which are both complex and complicated, and involve a clear understanding of both what you are trying to achieve through reflection and why you are trying to achieve it. In the following chapters of this book, we will address how reflective writing can be used within different contexts and practice roles to contribute to the ways in which advanced and expert practitioners work.

Further reading

The following provide further information: Alterio (2004); Blake (2005); Chirema (2007); Dye (2005); Grant, Kinnersley, Metcalf, Pill, and Houston (2006); Jasper (2008); Johns (2000); Simpson and Courtney (2007); Swindell and Watson (2006).

Reflective moment

Now turn back to the aims which you identified at the start of the chapter. To what extent have they been met? Write a paragraph outlining the factual and practical knowledge you have acquired through reading this chapter and doing the exercises. Write a second paragraph identifying any aims which you feel were only partially met or not met at all. As in previous chapters, divide your page into three columns. Head the first column 'What I need to learn', and make a list of any outstanding issues which you would like to learn more about. For example, you might wish to explore poetry as a form of reflective writing. Head the second column 'How I will learn it', and write down the ways in which your learning needs could be addressed; for example, through further reading, through attending study days, or through talking to other people. Head the third column 'How I will know that I have learnt it', and try to identify how you will know when you have met your needs.

6

Clinical supervision and reflective practice

Dawn Freshwater

Introduction

In this chapter we examine in more detail the interface between reflection, clinical supervision and reflective practice and discuss definitions and models for supervision and how these connect with reflection. We also look in-depth at the options for improving practice through reflection, clinical supervision and reflective practice using information, insights and ideas from practitioners involved in establishing clinical supervision in their respective areas. It is important to contextualize the discussion on reflection and clinical supervision prior to entering into any depth of debate. The idea of an individual wanting to make sense of the experiences they encounter is the point of departure, and is congruent with our particular ontological approach to reflection and clinical supervision, based on the assumption that an individual has an intrinsic desire to develop understanding and awareness. This process is the embodiment of work by many educationalists on dimensions of maturation, which is a key element of adult learning. However, when considering reflection and clinical supervision, two activities primarily concerned with development, we need to look critically at their relationship within the context of an adult learning from experience, and what it is we are attempting to achieve through their implementation.

Our aims for this chapter are:

1. to explore the relationship between clinical supervision and reflective practice;

2. to explore the assumptions, beliefs and values of both reflective practice and clinical supervision;
3. to discuss the impact that supervision might have on quality of care;
4. to outline and discuss the necessary conditions for effective clinical supervision; and
5. To help you to evaluate the role of clinical supervision in your current practice situation.

Reflective moment

Think carefully about our aims for Chapter 6. Now think about your own practice and how these aims might contribute towards developing it.

Based on our aims above, identify and write down some of your own, both in terms of what you hope to know and what you hope to be able to do after reading Chapter 6. We will return to these at the end of the chapter.

Reflection and clinical supervision

It is often assumed that reflective practice is at the heart of clinical supervision and is the foundation of what is sometimes termed guided reflection. Indeed, several authors note that clinical supervision involves critical reflection by the supervisee and the supervisor and as such provides an environment within which reflective practice can be fostered (Johns, 1993; Freshwater 2000; Rolfe et al., 2001; Johns and Freshwater, 2005). However, not all writers concur with the view that reflective practice is integral to clinical supervision, perhaps because the two concepts have been developed almost independently and as such have separate although interrelated evidence bases. Not surprisingly then, the discourse around clinical supervision and reflective practice is at times polarized and often confusing. As we have seen, one of the aims of this chapter is to further explore the assumptions, beliefs and values of both reflective practice and clinical supervision, in order to clarify how each refers and relates to the other.

We have already discussed various definitions of reflection, its processes and epistemology, and hence at this point it is sufficient to note that, from a health related perspective, reflection has been defined in different ways. Some definitions incorporate the product and the (often emancipatory) process envisaged by the author, whereas others frame reflection in terms of learning (Boud, Cohen and Walker, 2000; Jarvis, Holford and Griffin, 2001; Johns and Freshwater, 2005; Johns, 2006; Freshwater, 2007). Clinical supervision is described by numerous authors as being a structured system of reflection, primarily with the intention of improving practice (Driscoll, 2000; Spouse and Redfern, 2000; van Ooijen, 2003). An area that continues to be debated is that of the facilitation of reflective practice; just as practice cannot be changed in isolation, it is argued that practitioners struggle to objectify their own beliefs, values and actions without the benefit of another perspective. Burton (2000) argues that reflection needs to be guided and supported, referring to the earlier works of Johns (1996) and Cox, Hixon and Taylor (1991), and advocates the use of a skilled supervisor.

Reflective moment

Think about your own experiences of clinical supervision and reflective practice. How would you identify the relationship between them? What are your views about how clinical supervision may facilitate critical reflection?

Facilitating critical reflective practice through clinical supervision

It has been noted that there is a variety of ways in which the skills of critical reflection can be acquired, and that clinical supervision is one such way (Johns and Freshwater, 2005; Taylor, Kermode and Roberts, 2006). While clinical supervision is a fairly new concept in healthcare, it has a long tradition in such disciplines as counselling, psychotherapy, social work and midwifery. Rolfe et al. (2001) noted that initial interest in supervision in the UK developed as a direct result of two publications, these being *Vision for the Future* (Department of Health, 1993) and the position paper on clinical supervision commissioned by the Department of Health (Faugier and Butterworth, 1994). The United Kingdom Central Council for Nursing and Midwifery (UKCC, 1996) responded to these publications by highlighting the importance of adequate standards of supervision.

Clinical supervision is linked explicitly with practice development (UKCC, 1996), and appears to some extent to have been reified as the ideal forum within which to foster reflective practice. While it would not be true to say that all the literature around clinical supervision emphasizes the skills of reflection, it is fair to say that the two concepts are often described concurrently. Many models of clinical supervision have been presented, nearly all of which include an element of reflection and reflective practice (Holloway, 1995; Bond and Holland, 1998; Hawkins and Shohet, 2006), while others suggest reflection is itself a model for supervision (Todd and Freshwater, 1999; Johns, 2000; Van Ooijen, 2000; Rolfe et al. 2001; Johns and Freshwater, 2005). In addition, some of the most widely used definitions of clinical supervision make reflective practice central to their aims.

Definitions of clinical supervision abound; put simply, clinical supervision can be described as a flexible and dynamic structure within which to continuously deconstruct and reconstruct clinical practice. Fundamental to this process of deconstruction and reconstruction are the skills of reflection, critical reflection and reflexivity. In other words, clinical supervision and reflective practice are interdependent and inextricably linked through the process of reflection. Allied health professionals and nurses alike have embraced this approach to clinical supervision as an instrument to improve practice, and in some cases supervision has been accentuated by including it in official publications of professional statutory bodies (NMC, 2002). The Department of Health (1993), now some 17 years ago, defined clinical supervision as:

A term to describe a formal process of professional support and learning which enables practitioners to develop knowledge and competence, assume responsibility for their own practice and enhance consumer protection and safety of care in complex situations.

More recently, and in an updated text, Bishop (2006, p. 17) focused on the interactional aspects of clinical supervision, suggesting that supervision is:

A designated interaction between two or more practitioners within a safe and supportive environment, that enables a continuum of reflective, critical analysis of care, to ensure quality patient services, and the well-being of the practitioner.

In contrast to the published definitions above, a working definition suggested by a group of experienced multi-professional practitioners during a training programme on clinical supervision after they had critically discussed the evolved definitions (ALG, 2006) is stated as:

> A time-protected interaction between two or more professionals in a safe, supportive and confidential environment to discuss, reflect and critically analyze work issues. The aim of clinical support is to encourage self-development and improve work practices.

As always, comparing definitions provides some interesting points for discussion. The practitioners' definition illustrates their understanding of the limited resources in 'real life', as they put it, in which they accentuate the need for protected time. In this small scale, but national, study of the implementation of clinical supervision within secure environments, this was one of the most important issues raised as influencing the successful implementation, and importantly, sustainability of clinical supervision within specific departments. A further element included in the practitioners' definition is the focus on discussing *work issues* to improve practice, while also attending to and articulating the importance of individual development.

An additional observation is the fact that both the Department of Health (1993) and Bishop (2006) suggest clinical supervision as *enabling* practitioners to ensure high quality care. This illuminates two points for discussion. The first point to highlight is the use of the word *enable*. Espeland and Shanta (2001) discuss the dichotomy of enabling versus empowering and quote Haber et al. (1997) as defining enabling as 'behaviours by others that perpetuates dependent behaviours'. This is contrary to the idea of an adult striving for self-actualization and personal development. More specifically, it conflicts with authors who consider reflective processes to be transformational for the individual (Johns and Freshwater, 2005). Bishop's (2006) interpretation of *enable*, within the context of her definition, appears to relate to the process of analysis itself being enabled rather than the practitioner, although this is, in itself, open to interpretation. One might ask whether reflection and clinical supervision should not focus on emancipating the practitioner, which would, as a result, enable them to analyze their practice critically. Of course, both the process of analysis and practitioner development are interrelated and, as such, it is perhaps not entirely necessary to foreground either the personal development and emancipation of the practitioner or the liberation of an analytic process, when one is so dependant on the other. Suffice it to say that supervision is one way of providing an environment for analytic processes and personal development through reflection to be enhanced and facilitated.

The second point to be highlighted here, which can be developed from the discussion on the semantics of *enabling* versus *emancipation*, is the concept of power and control. Gilbert (2001), for example, suggests that clinical supervision can be seen as a form of surveillance in which organizations are able to establish formal structures for exercising control. The definition used by the Department of Health (1993), in which clinical supervision enables the practitioner to *assume responsibility*, implies that this is not happening and the idea of surveillance becomes more tangible when the responsibility to establish supervision is delegated to a local level where the reality is that line managers supervise their staff. Although Bishop (2006) appears to suggest *enabling* rather than *empowering* practitioners, she also highlights the organizational influence and suggests, among other things, that a governmental preoccupation with audit and evidence-based practice could move the focus of clinical supervision away from the philosophical development of individual practitioners towards a method of ensuring standards of quality are being met. Within this context, Bishop, we feel, underpins the notion of wanting to enable the practitioner to develop a *process* of critical thought in her definition. The idea of enabling a process has a different weight from the Department of Health definition, which suggests incapability. What we can begin to see here is a potential polarized view of clinical supervision, one which places the process of critical reflection at one end of the continuum, and the issues of surveillance, monitoring and Big Brother type accountability at the other end. Simply put, there is a discrepancy between the positioning of power and authority, who owns it, and who has the authority to act in any given practical situation. We would argue that clinical supervision is concerned with both the process of critical reflection, which by definition, includes an element of acting in good faith, and with using power, knowledge and autonomy effectively and with consideration. (See Chapter 2 for a further discussion on power and knowledge.)

In other aspects, the definition by Bishop (2006) and the one put forward by the practitioners are comparable in their attention to personal development and quality of care. There is, however, another area of debate, namely that of the nomenclature. Numerous practitioners question the relevance of *clinical* supervision and this terminology results in confusion and frustration as it implies that supervisory sessions may only be used to discuss patient-related, clinical issues. There are of course many other issues influencing

Figure 6.1 Professional development as the common theme between reflective practice, reflection and clinical supervision

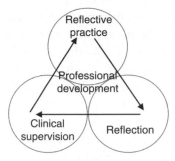

the individual practitioner's professional development; not least of all, issues relating to management, inter-professional interaction, relationships with peers and patients' families and organizational concerns.

To this end, Esterhuizen and Freshwater (2008) examined the connection between clinical supervision, reflection and reflective practice in more detail. In their view, it is the relationship between reflection and clinical supervision that results in reflective practice (see Figure 6.1). They claim that 'reflection is a cyclic thought process (a skill) and clinical supervision is a method that can be used to focus and guide the individual's reflective process (a structure), the change that arises from this contextualised, analytical, process results in reflective practice (a way of being)' (Esterhuizen and Freshwater, 2008). They interestingly point to the observation by Driscoll (2000), who suggests that 'Not all reflective practice is clinical supervision but potentially all good clinical supervision is reflective practice'.

Clinical supervision, then, when well facilitated, can provide cues for reflection allowing the individual to identify their own ways of knowing. In our experience of working with groups, whether this be through group supervision (see Chapter 7) or through more informal teaching and learning processes, ways of knowing are always just below the surface. The science (empirics) and the art (aesthetics) of caring, the ethics of care and personal knowledge are usually extracted during discussions, often initiated by the group members and practitioners themselves, without too much interference from the facilitator. It is not necessarily the case that practitioners categorize or classify their thinking according to a particular knowledge framework (such as, for example, Carper's work on nursing), but in addressing ways of knowing through the content of discussions, practitioners are able to recognize and understand the components of being which assist us in self awareness, furthering development and providing a foothold towards the elusive concept of self-actualization, or perhaps more specifically, to understand and reach our personal potential in professional development. In essence, we are referring here to the therapeutic nature of clinical supervision and reflective practice, something that has been the subject of, and debated in, much health care literature.

Reflective moment

How often do you share your thoughts and experiences of professional practice with others? Identify both formal and informal situations in which this process takes place.

Spend some time thinking about the benefits of reflecting on your practice with the guidance of another professional. Perhaps you can think of a specific time when you have talked to someone about a particular work situation. Did this help, and if so, how? Write a paragraph outlining what you think you gain from sharing your practice with another person. Also make a note of any concerns that come to mind.

Write a brief paragraph stating what you want from clinical supervision. Now complete the following statements, clarifying as many of your hopes, expectations and fears as you are able at this time.

- When I come to supervision I hope I will...
- I expect I will...
- I am afraid I will...

Reflection, clinical supervision and reflective practice are bound together by a common focus and, as such, interrelate. However, in some circumstances they function independently inasmuch as an individual may have internalized elements of their professional role to the degree that they do not need to reflect actively and consciously, as in the case of the expert practitioner (Benner's early work of 1984 is a good example of this, and is discussed further in Chapter 8). In a different situation, the same individual may feel the need to reflect on a specific element of care in order to internalize it, and in yet another situation they may feel the need for facilitated clinical supervision in order to analyze and understand the implications of a situation, prior to or building on private reflection and incorporation into their scope of practice as a reflective practitioner. When viewed from this perspective, reflection and clinical supervision combine to produce a reflective practitioner embodying reflective practice.

Clinical supervision as a tool for personal development

When facilitating participants across disciplines in clinical supervision programmes it becomes apparent that, although the individual's development as a professional is the focus, it also impacts on their personal development. It is therefore important to keep clinical supervision grounded in their daily work and discipline.

There is a definite tension between accepting and understanding the holistic nature of the individual practitioner, knowing that reflections and awareness in a professional domain will have an impact on their personal life, and accepting and understanding the individual's attempts to maintain a boundary between personal and professional aspects of their life. The early but enduring work of Bond and Holland (1998) focuses on professional development, but the same principle can, of course, be transferred by the individual to other areas of their life (see Table 6.1).

As it is impossible for an individual to prevent awareness and insight in their professional behaviour from impacting on their personal lives and visa versa, it is important to remain mindful of this phenomenon and to maintain a healthy division between (clinical) supervision related to professional issues and counselling on a more personal level (Driscoll, 2000). As such, parties need to be aware that any issue an individual needs to reflect on from a professional perspective generally has a personal component that may need to be addressed. Alternatively, behaviour manifesting in a professional setting will often be identified by the individual as occurring in their personal lives too. Realizing and respecting this interface between personal and professional is, for us, the essence of developing self-awareness as an individual in order to adapt behaviour and ultimately change or improve practice.

Van Ooijen (2003), in her book on clinical supervision, distinguishes between counselling as developing *a greater personal awareness of one's inner landscape*, and supervision as focusing on work. In general, authors writing on this subject are clear that, while being

Table 6.1 Differences between counselling and clinical supervision

	Counselling	Clinical supervision
Agenda	Agenda defined by the supervisee	Agenda mostly defined by the supervisee. Clinical supervisor may add items arising during the sessions or refocus on how any personal issues discussed affect practice.
Confidentiality	Total, with legal exceptions. Counsellor or client may keep own records that are absolutely confidential.	Almost total, with exceptions of legal or professional ethics. Record may be made to pass on within the organization of attendance dates and times. Record of content may be negotiated between practitioner and clinical supervisor, for their eyes only.
Information from facilitator	Information, advice or guidance very rarely given, and then usually focused on emotional issues.	Some information, advice, guidance offered to supplement the supervisee's own expertise, to help the supervisee see options available and make their own informed decision.
Challenge from facilitator	Non-judgmental about the person's emotional issues. Very occasional challenges about defences against emotional expression and growth.	Challenging technical mistakes, inadequate clinical standards, and contribution to problems with team work, more personal issues such as unhelpful or self-defeating behaviours or attitudes, blind spots, broken contracts. Based on evidence gained during the clinical supervision session.
Support from facilitator	Support for the client as a person, often especially for emotional awareness and expression. Support is open-ended.	Support for the supervisee as a person and encouragement given to help supervisee recognize and use own expertise and personal abilities towards developing their professional expertise. Any exploration of personal issues is eventually related back to how these affect practice. Clinical supervisor acknowledges any emotional issues about the past which are disclosed, but suggests that his/her remit is to help with the present-day feelings and practicalities.
Catalytic help from facilitator	Enabling reflection and problem solving in the direction of deeper exploration into the personal and relationship aspects of the problem, including the transference relationship between client and counsellor.	Enabling reflection on issues ultimately affecting practice (including some consideration of issues involved in the clinical supervision relationship), learning from experience, problem solving, pinpointing ways of dealing with difficult emotions, decision making and planning. All of these with the ultimate emphasis on reviewing application to practice.

Source: Adapted from Bond and Holland (1998, p. 134).

aware of the overlap between counselling and supervision, all parties have a responsibility to identify and maintain clear boundaries when personal issues manifest themselves. The supervisor has the explicit responsibility to maintain her role, and both Driscoll and Van Ooijen support the principle that the supervisee should address any specific, personal, issue – but in a different setting. As part of her role, the supervisor could suggest where the individual may receive help, but should in no way take on the role of counsellor. Given the potentially confusing interface between counselling and supervision, one option in maintaining clarity could be to set specific goals for each supervisory session in which the focus of the session is articulated.

Over two decades ago, Proctor (1986) suggested a model and framework of supervision that could be beneficial in helping the supervisee to set an agenda and maintain the necessary focus. This model is still a useful practical tool for applying and understanding some of the essential components of clinical supervision, and as such we include an adapted version here (see Figure 6.2).

It is clear from Proctor's model that any supervision session will incorporate not only the three functions mentioned here (although often one is more predominant), but of course many more aspects, such as ways of knowing and levels of reflection.

Figure 6.2 Three functions of Proctor's interactive model of supervision

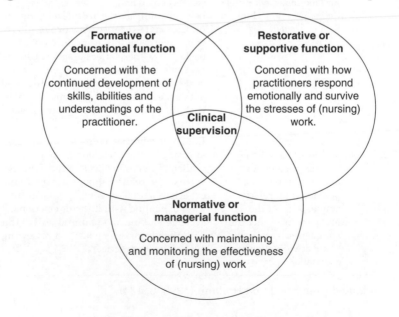

Formative or educational function

Concerned with the continued development of skills, abilities and understandings of the practitioner.

Restorative or supportive function

Concerned with how practitioners respond emotionally and survive the stresses of (nursing) work.

Clinical supervision

Normative or managerial function

Concerned with maintaining and monitoring the effectiveness of (nursing) work

Using Proctor's model to support a supervisee to analyze the focus they want supervision to have prior to the session and evaluating at the end whether this was, in fact, the most appropriate choice, could provide the supervisee with a practical, transferable skill of being able to recognize an issue and focus on it during personal reflection. Of course, this begins to take the individual practitioner to the critical edge of reflection.

Finally, when considering personal and professional boundaries in supervision, we would do well to remember that reflection or clinical supervision on professional issues, while important, is *one* part of the larger picture for the individual. Professional investment is but one section of the individual's life and not the other way around. Retaining this principle could also help the supervisee to maintain perspective on professional situations and could be helpful in setting boundaries for both supervisee and supervisor.

The importance of practice in clinical supervision

As we have already indicated with Proctor's work, we think it is important that a practitioner maintains the focus on practice-related situations during supervision. Freshwater (2007) refers to the work

Figure 6.3 Quality of care as the focus of clinical supervision

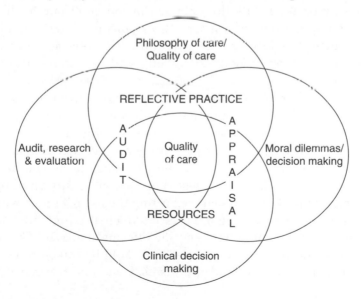

of Donald Schön and suggests the importance of reflecting on experience in order to contextualize the situation and therefore to learn from it.

Esterhuizen and Freshwater (2008) identify a further way of supporting a practitioner to reflect on a clinical role, which is to incorporate the four different aspects of the role as a means of approaching and analyzing a practice-related situation they wish to discuss during supervision (see Figure 6.3).

There is no specific direction from which to analyze a situation; a practitioner can approach her analysis from whichever perspective she considers to be the most appropriate or to have the greatest priority.

Using this type of approach provides neutrality for the practitioner and, although the discussion focuses on her specific issues, the model can make allowances for structure and a feeling of *objectivity,* which may make supervision less threatening to the individual. Clinical supervision sessions focussing on the quality of care can be used equally effectively for individual and group supervision, the latter having the advantage of providing a shared learning experience among colleagues (see Chapter 7).

Quality of care is, of course, a multi-faceted concept, and is linked to competencies, and as Gilbert (2001) suggests, clinical supervision could potentially become a method of surveillance. However, Clouder and Sellars (2004) suggest that there may be a case for using clinical supervision as a means of surveillance, considering the miscarriage of ethics by professionals throughout the course of our health care history. Organizations are, after all, responsible for the quality of care provided. Even though individual practitioners are responsible for their actions, any negative publicity will be detrimental to the organization.

The implication of providing facilitated supervision is an expensive commodity for an organization, and it could be argued that managers should have some idea as to what is being discussed during supervisory sessions, and that practitioners have a responsibility to provide transparency as to what they consider to be the benefits. Clouder and Sellars (2004) suggest that a possible way forward is to be explicit (rather than implicit) regarding the use of clinical supervision as a means of obtaining information to ensure high quality care and provide management with specific information. While Northcott (2000) suggests that clinical supervision could be linked to performance management and annual appraisals, Pesut and Herman's (1999)

Figure 6.4 The intent-emphasis grid

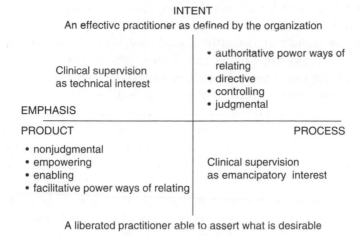

Source: Adapted from Johns (2001).

work on clinical reasoning illustrates how client-related decision making could be incorporated into supervisory sessions. It is hard to support the idea of clinical supervision being used as a method of control and management; nevertheless some do defend this position.

Johns (2001) illustrates the emancipating versus controlling use of clinical supervision and seems to suggest a polarization related to the intention of the supervisor (Figure 6.4).

There continue to be questions regarding the issue of who should facilitate reflection through clinical supervision, that is to say, who should or can be a clinical supervisor. Van Ooijen (2003) suggests that the practitioner could benefit from supervision by an outsider and a manager. In some ways this can also be a weakness if, as Van Ooijen goes on to suggest, this form of managerial supervision is dependent on the relationship between the parties being balanced and affable. The construction of managerial supervision may create complications if some staff chose managerial supervision while others chose to have clinical supervision from an outsider. Although both methods could result in practitioners learning and developing, it is feasible that it could create discrepancies between staff members within a team. The potential difference between managerial and outside facilitation could lie in the terminology: coaching versus clinical supervision. It would be ill-advised to introduce another term for an intervention unless it is clear to all parties what the difference is.

Coaching could be undertaken by the unit manager to support individual development towards an agreed point: a team vision/ philosophy including specific knowledge and skills (Spouse and Redfern, 2000; Boud, Cohen and Walker, 2000), whereas an external facilitator could provide clinical supervision to support personal development. Specific terminology for specific interventions focused on achieving particular objectives is necessary to provide clarity between the roles. Creating an opportunity for structured reflection, facilitated by an outsider and as a form of managerial support by way of coaching, would provide an opening for development and growth on the part of the practitioner *and* the chance for the line manager to meet with their staff and obtain insight about development towards achieving objectives as defined by the team.

It could be argued that the supervisee's experience of supervision is heavily dependant upon the orientation of the facilitator. Lahteenmaki (2005) observes that the supervision that students receive is closely related to their supervisor's view of the goals of learning, and other writers concur with this view (see, for example, Van Ooijen, 2003). For example, in the apprentice – master approach to learning, which relies heavily on the technical instrumental philosophy of education, the supervisee/practitioner is viewed as a passive recipient of knowledge. By way of contrast, reflective and critical approaches to learning, which emphasize the role of the supervisee/ practitioner in analyzing and understanding their own practices, concentrate on eliciting the supervisee's espoused theories and values. As with all learning situations, some individuals respond better to the apprentice – master approach to learning, finding reflection threatening and challenging, most often because it forces them to reflect on and develop an inner authority through the constant testing of personal and relational hypotheses. Most experienced facilitators of learning would point out that the real skill of supervision is in integrating facilitative and directive skills to enable an optimal learning environment to suit the individual needs of the practitioner/ learner.

We have discussed the concept of clinical supervision as a method of improving practice, and/or ensuring best practice, but have also pointed out its potential to be used as a means of control and surveillance. Clinical supervision is, we have argued, work-related and is fundamentally aimed at improving practice and developing the individual. The focus of supervision is practice-based, whatever that practice, allowing for exploration of the personal domain but always returning to the work-related topic incorporating any new insights.

Further reading

We have cited a great number of authors in our discussion of reflective practice and clinical supervision. If you wish to be more selective in your reading, you might wish to begin with the following: Clouder and Sellars (2004); Lahteenmaki (2005); Jasper (2006); Johns (2009); Johns and Freshwater (2005).

The supervisory relationship

It is widely accepted that the success of clinical supervision is highly dependant on the quality and effectiveness of the supervisory relationship (Kohner, 1994). In addition, as we have already indicated, there is a prevalent view that the supervisor should not be the supervisee's manager, although we have also cited some arguments in its favour, and on occasions it might in any case be difficult to avoid. So who can be your supervisor? A supervisor might be a peer, a more experienced professional, an external facilitator, or a manager who is not directly responsible to you, but should be someone who shares a similar vision to yours of the intent and emphasis of clinical supervision (Johns, 1998).

Reflective moment

With a colleague, spend some time discussing the advantages and disadvantages of the following:

● Individual supervision;
● Group supervision;
● Peer supervision;
● Managerial supervision;
● Multidisciplinary supervision; and
● Supervision with an allocated supervisor.

How do you choose your supervisor? If you go back to the previous exercises in this chapter, in which you explored what has been helpful for you in the past when you have been supervised and your list of hopes, expectations and fears about supervision, you might find that these will help to identify the sort of person you are looking for. Ideally, this should be someone who can offer you challenge as much as support, someone you feel you can work with personally and professionally, whom you have respect for, and who can help you to develop in areas that you know are lacking. Often, someone from a different discipline can help you to see things from a wider perspective by challenging the embedded norms of your everyday practice. Other points that may influence your choice of supervisor might be age, gender and cultural factors. Choosing the person you would want to be your supervisor is important, but there are also practical issues to consider such as convenient timing, shift patterns, appropriate venues and your willingness to be flexible. Where possible, we would suggest that you find a venue for your supervision which is away from your usual work area, and where you are less likely to be interrupted and perhaps able to speak more freely. However, if this is not practical, it is important to find an environment within which you feel safe. When choosing your supervisor it is worth bearing in mind their training and experience and any specific interests they carry which will act as a background to the work you do together.

Reflective moment

Take some time now to think about supervision you have experienced in the past, whether this has been formally labelled 'clinical' supervision, or has involved some other sort of supervisory relationship, such as being mentored, or within preceptorship.

Did you have choice of a supervisor?

What type of relationship did you have with your supervisor?

What were the positive aspects that your supervisor brought to the relationship?

Were there any areas of supervision which you feel could have been more effective?

What features would you look for next time you are looking for a supervisor?

Another influence on your decision is what particular mode of supervision you would prefer, given that you have a choice. When selecting a particular form of supervision, it is important that you are clear about what is available, who makes the decision, and how and why it is made.

Modes of supervision

The literature often presents conflicting and confusing ideas about the modes and models of clinical supervision. The *model* of supervision refers to the theoretical and philosophical underpinnings of supervision and the way in which this informs the work, and these issues will be discussed later in the chapter. The *mode* of clinical supervision refers to the practical ways of operationalizing the process itself, such as individual, group, peer or managerial supervision. There are benefits and limitations to each mode of supervision, both for the individual and for the organization.

Organizations often prefer groups for reasons of efficacy and cost effectiveness, and this is something that will be addressed in detail when we outline the theory and practice of group supervision in Chapter 7. However, individual or one-to-one supervision is often the first choice for beginning supervisees, especially those who experience difficulty with self-disclosure or find groups threatening. One-to-one supervision has the benefits of allowing the supervisor and supervisee not only to concentrate their attentions on the development of the working alliance, but also has the added advantage of giving the supervisee more time.

In contrast, peer supervision emphasizes the role of self and peer assessment as a resource for ongoing professional development. A peer group is one that consists of people who judge themselves to be at an equal level to each other, and in which all members of the group are supervisees and supervisors, all are deemed competent, and where feedback is based on shared expertise and collaborative partnerships in what might be termed a hierarchy among equals (Heron 1981; Bond and Holland, 1998). Peer supervision may also take the form of one-to-one supervision in which the time is shared between the two individuals. A list of the key characteristics of individual, group and peer supervision is outlined below.

Individual

- This form of supervision has the advantage of the continuity and intimacy of the one-to-one relationship which may enhance the professional development of the practitioner.
- The process and feedback inevitably depends upon the supervisor's style, ethical and theoretical preferences.
- Feedback will be limited to that of the supervisor. An issue for the supervisee is how to compensate for this bias, and to that end

the supervisor's task is to encourage the supervisee to use a broad range of additional professional resources.

Group

- Case material can be used in such a way that provides a learning opportunity for the whole group.
- It is crucial to the function of the group to establish ground rules and to discuss equal access to supervision.
- There is potential for the group to be used as a resource for feedback processes and the creation of a variety of perspectives.
- The size of the group can affect the success of the supervision.

Peer

- Supervision acts as a resource for ongoing professional development and support.
- It is based on mutual feedback and shared expertise.
- It provides a hierarchy among equals through collaborative partnerships.

Having decided upon a mode of supervision which is both agreeable and practical, it is important to ascertain a framework within which you and your supervisor can work. There are many models of supervision that you may wish to explore with your supervisor, which were discussed in the first edition of this book (Rolfe et al., 2001), and which can be accessed through the Guides to further reading.

Frameworks of supervision

The frameworks for supervision fall broadly into three categories: structural, developmental and goal-oriented.

Structural frameworks

The cyclic model developed for counselling by Page and Woskett (1994) provides a structured sequential model with five phases, each subdivided into a further five (see Figure 6.5). This comprehensive model provides the supervisor with a flexible set of guidelines which are designed to be used in an integrative way as opposed to a rigid framework to be adhered to. The guidelines enable the supervisor to develop personally and the supervisee in a professional manner, viewing the

Figure 6.5 A sequential model of supervision

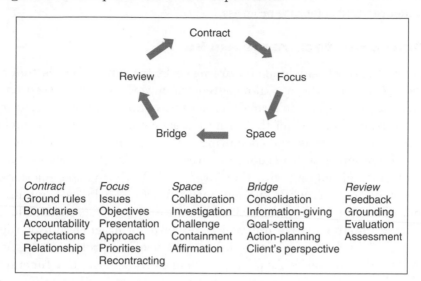

Contract	Focus	Space	Bridge	Review
Ground rules	Issues	Collaboration	Consolidation	Feedback
Boundaries	Objectives	Investigation	Information-giving	Grounding
Accountability	Presentation	Challenge	Goal-setting	Evaluation
Expectations	Approach	Containment	Action-planning	Assessment
Relationship	Priorities	Affirmation	Client's perspective	
	Recontracting			

Source: Adapted from Page and Woskett (1994).

supervision process as one of dynamic movement rather than being static, with change regarded as fundamental both to the practice of supervision and to clinical practice.

As we can see, each of the five phases in this framework offers guidance as to how to conduct a supervision session, making explicit the necessary tasks. This structural type of approach can be very helpful for the beginning supervisor and, indeed, for the novice supervisee. Many frameworks of reflection are presented in a cyclical format (see Chapter 3), and can therefore run parallel to Page and Woskett's (1994) structural framework of supervision.

Developmental frameworks

Developmental approaches originate in developmental psychology, and not surprisingly they emphasize the educational functions of clinical supervision, moving from the child through the adolescent and young adult to maturity (Stoltenberg and Delworth, 1987). In these approaches, the supervisee is seen to move from a place of felt novice to perceived expert during the course of her supervision (Benner, 1984).

Hawkins and Shohet's (2006) process framework is one such developmental approach, in which emphasis is placed on the development of the supervisory alliance as a way of encouraging and empowering the supervisee. This framework is helpful in enabling the practitioner to identify and celebrate progress.

Goal-oriented frameworks

One of the most widely quoted frameworks for supervision is that of Proctor (1986), whose goal-oriented framework was discussed earlier, and focuses on the formative, normative and restorative tasks of supervision. The task of the formative educational function includes monitoring, teaching and consulting for lifelong learning and professional development. The supportive restorative function involves containment and holding with the purpose of alleviating the emotional labour of practice, while the normative function includes examining the organizational issues, including ethical dimensions, the code of practice, administrative functions, standards of practice and quality control. This framework is useful in that it offers professional guidance (in the normative function), challenge (in the formative function) and support (in the restorative function), hence recognizing the need for balance between these elements. As with the models discussed earlier, all of the above frameworks have something to offer the supervisory alliance, and the flexible practitioner will be able to utilize and adapt aspects of several frameworks within a dynamic situation such as supervision. What all the frameworks have in common is the requirement for self-reflection and developing self-awareness as part of becoming a reflective and effective practitioner.

One well-known framework that encompasses this notion of becoming self-aware in practice is the Johari window. As can be seen from Figure 6.6, our awareness is expanded as we take the risk of disclosing some of our 'hidden' areas and by being receptive to feedback from others about our 'blind spots'. For this level of self-disclosure to occur

Figure 6.6 Clinical supervision and the Johari window

	Known to self	Not known to self
Known to others	Open self Increased via clinical supervision	Blind self Discovered via clinical supervision
Not known to others	Hidden self Revealed and explored via trust and confidence in clinical supervision	Unknown self Decreased via clinical supervision

Source: Adapted from Heath and Freshwater (2000), via Lufe (1969).

there need to be certain boundaries in place to ensure the safety and trust of the supervisee. It is essential that these boundaries are discussed in the first session of supervision as part of the contractual negotiation.

Contracting

In setting up clinical supervision, it is essential that the boundaries of the supervisory relationship are established through the explicit drawing-up of ground rules via a mutually negotiated contract. The contract is made as explicit as possible between all interested parties, not only to encourage ownership but also to allow individuals to make an informed choice about the relationship they are embarking on. This initial session is also helpful in encouraging individual practitioners to reflect upon their beliefs, needs and values, so the process of reflection begins immediately.

What would you need to have in place in order to embark upon a supervisory alliance?

Make a list of items that you would want to discuss with your supervisor/supervisee when negotiating your working contract.

Some of the things you might want to consider in negotiating a clear contract include:

- openness on both sides;
- preparation requirements (i.e what does the supervisor expect you to do prior to a supervisory session?);
- awareness of the value of supervision as a resource;
- development of good working skills as the most important aim of the relationship;
- focus (which is always the working effectiveness of the supervisee);
- accountability;
- responsibility of the supervisor;
- awareness of supervisee's level;
- agreement on needs and appropriate material; and
- practical matters including time boundaries, venue and confidentiality.

Confidentiality is something that often concerns supervisees. This is not surprising, since we have already seen that there is considerable confusion around the differences and similarities between supervision, line management and professional discussion with colleagues.

The dynamics of the supervisory relationship

The role of the supervisor

Many writers have attempted to detail the fundamental features of the role of the supervisor (Faugier, 1992; Faugier and Butterworth, 1994; Johns and McCormack, 1998; Fitzgerald, 2000). Importance is usually placed on the supervisor having a willingness to facilitate learning in others while being open to learning about themselves, and it is thought to be essential that supervisors have a willingness to undertake self-assessment and that they should not only have training in supervision but should also be in supervision themselves (Kohner, 1994). This is crucial if the supervisor is going to role model one of the fundamental purposes of supervision to the supervisee, that is, to look at the intention behind the intervention. Some authors are of the opinion that many of the skills required for the role of clinical supervisor can be equated with the skills of the effective practitioner (Johns, 1998; Fowler, 1996).

Reflective moment

Looking back at your previous writing which identifies your hopes, expectations and fears regarding clinical supervision, think about choosing your own ideal supervisor. Discuss with a colleague the specific skills and qualities of the ideal supervisor.

Now spend some time together reflecting on these qualities and the ways in which you meet them.

The supervisor's preferred relationship model, her definition of supervision and her supervisory styles heavily influence the role of the supervisor, as we can see from the styles described below:

Constructive
The supervisor is very helpful, which has obvious benefits in the early stages of supervision, but if continued this style can eventually lead to the supervisee feeling smothered. When using the developmental approach, the supervisor needs to be aware of when it is appropriate to allow the supervisee to walk on her own even if there is a risk of falling.

Authoritative

The supervisee feels that their work is constantly under a microscope, and experiences the supervisor as picky. The supervisor may recognize that they have perfectionist tendencies which might be useful at times, especially when considering the normative function of supervision, but may be off putting in the early stages of supervision when the task is to build a safe trusting relationship. This style can be linked to managerial supervision.

Didactic/consultative

The supervisor focuses on the educational components of information-giving and providing the supervisee with the benefit of wisdom and experience. Again, this can be very important at all stages of the supervisory work and is especially helpful at the beginning for the novice supervisor. However, the supervisor can forget that the supervisee is also a teacher and has wisdom. This style might be likened to mentorship/preceptorship.

Amorphous

The supervisor is not really present for the supervisee, she is without shape and appears invisible in her interventions. The supervisee can feel unsupported and unheard due to a lack of boundaries; developmentally the supervisee needs to be held and contained. Perhaps the first phase of Page and Woskett's (1994) framework has not been established, and the relationship is missing. However, it can sometimes be important for the supervisor to be more in the background, especially when the supervisee is sophisticated, although the supervisor would usually be making a conscious choice to hold back.

Unsupportive

The supervisor is present but offers little or no supportive interventions; challenges are cold and punitive with a hint of authority about them. Challenge is important but the timeliness of interventions is crucial and always in relation to the stage of the supervisory alliance. Unfortunately, this style of supervision can feel too much like clinical practice to the practitioner, where she is often left feeling unsupported.

Therapeutic

The supervisor concentrates on the personal needs of the supervisee, moving into a counselling role and overstepping boundaries. There is a fine line between this style and Proctor's (1986) restorative function, and while therapeutic input can be part of the work, the boundaries between counselling, therapy and supervision need to be made clear.

Detective

This style of supervision focuses on trying to find the cause of problems and lay blame. The supervisor feels that they have to get to the bottom of things and understand the complete story, hence detail is important. The supervisee can feel like they are under oath and under investigation.

Reflective/facilitative

The reflective supervisor draws upon a facilitative style that incorporates personal experience and insight but that also permits inclusion as a professional learner. Interventions are supportive, including the use of feelings and cognitions, but are also probing and challenging. Some of the skills of the effective reflective supervisor are outlined below.

Skills of reflective supervision

The effective reflective supervisor knows when it is appropriate to make a particular type of intervention using:

Listening and responding skills

- Ability to use various forms of questions to elicit further information and to stimulate reflection.
- Ability to respond to the supervisee using a variety of skills including clarifying, summarizing, reflecting and accepting.
- Ability to use clear questions focused on the supervisee's professional context.

Reflexive skills

- The ability to recognize your own skills and the impact that these have on the supervisory interaction, which presupposes a certain degree of self-awareness.
- The ability to check your own ideas, preconceptions and hypotheses and the effect of these on supervision.
- The ability to evaluate the effects of your approach to supervision on the supervisee and the supervisory relationship.
- The ability to be flexible in your approach to supervisory methods, style or mode in order to be a more effective supervisor.

Observing skills

- Recognizing progress and acknowledging it with the supervisee.
- Identifying areas for further development.
- Observing the strengths and weaknesses of the supervisee and of the supervisory relationship.
- Noticing recurrent themes or patterns in your work with the supervisee and between the supervisee and their clinical practice.

Transparency

- The skills to use self-disclosure appropriately.
- The ability to be open about your way of working.
- Being open about your own opinion without imposing it on the supervisee.
- Being able to justify reasons for interventions made.
- Ability to reflect openly on the specific emphasis of supervision.

Feedback

- Being able to stay with the supervisee's fear and anxieties.
- Ability to give positive feedback without appearing patronizing.
- Responding to the supervisee in a non-judgmental manner based on the belief that the supervisee is acting in the best way she can at that moment and is also willing to learn.

Sensitivity to wider social issues

- Being aware of and being able to respond sensitively to power differentials.
- Being aware of the social context within which the supervisee is operating and the influence of this on the supervisory relationship.
- The ability to stimulate the development of the supervisee's skills within the working context.
- Noticing the influence of the supervisee's social background, belief systems, norms and values on the supervisory relationship and the wider working context.

Creativity and flexibility

- The skills to be able to create and offer a variety of different methods and techniques for reflection.

It would be impossible for every supervisor to achieve every skill on this list in every session of supervision, and it is important for the supervisor to acknowledge that they are also in the constant process of reflection-on-action and, as such, aspires to be what Winnicott (1971) might have termed the 'good enough supervisor' (Heath and Freshwater, 2000).

The role of the supervisee

The supervisory alliance also makes certain demands of the supervisee, who also requires skills to fulfil her responsibilities. Supervisees are required to be proactive in the relationship and to realize that they have an equal part in monitoring and evaluating the supervisory alliance (Kohner, 1994). In preparation for supervision, the practitioner is expected to reflect upon practice incidents prior to the session, perhaps doing a 'mini-supervision' through critical reflection to sharpen her awareness of the issues for discussion. This not only encourages the supervisee to develop the skills of reflection-on-action, but also gives the responsibility for setting the supervisory agenda to the supervisee, so that the available time can be used to best advantage.

Supervisees can engage in a variety of exercises to enhance their capacity to adequately prepare for supervision, some of which you have been doing as you have moved through this text, such as reflective writing, using a model of reflection, and gathering further information to inform your decision-making.

Reflective moment

Now turn back to the aims you identified at the start of the chapter. To what extent have they been met? Write a paragraph outlining the factual and practical knowledge you have acquired through reading this chapter and doing the exercises. Write a second paragraph identifying any aims which you feel were only partially met or not met at all. As in previous chapters, divide your page into three columns. Head the first column 'What I need to learn', and make a list of any outstanding issues which you would like to learn more about. For example, you might wish to explore further some of the frameworks for supervision mentioned earlier. Head the second column 'How I will learn it', and write down the ways in which your learning needs could be addressed; for example, through further reading, through attending study days, or through talking to other people. Head the third column 'How I will know that I have learnt it', and try to identify how you will know when you have met your needs.

7

Group supervision

Gary Rolfe

Introduction

While many managers and practitioners are fully aware of the benefits of supervision and wish to introduce it into their practice areas, they are often hampered by a lack of resources, including insufficient time, not enough trained and experienced supervisors, and a shortage of money to pay for outside supervision. The solution that more and more individuals and organizations are turning to is some form of group supervision.

We have already discussed the principles of supervision in some depth, and so in this chapter we will focus on groups and the particular issues involved in supervising and being supervised in group settings. Our aim is therefore to enable you to learn more about the theory and practice of group supervision, and in particular to reflect on your experience of being in groups of all kinds. More specifically, our aims for this chapter are:

1　to explore the benefits and disadvantages of supervision in groups;
2　to help you to reflect on your experiences in groups from a variety of different theoretical perspectives;
3　to enable you to plan and organize a supervision group;
4　to enable you to reflect on your personal attributes as a group facilitator; and
5　to outline and discuss the basic skills required to safely and competently begin facilitating a supervision group.

Reflective moment

Think carefully about our aims for Chapter 7. Now think about your own practice and how these aims might contribute towards developing it.

Based on our aims above, identify write down some aims of your own, both in terms of what you hope to know and what you hope to be able to do after reading Chapter 7. We will return to these at the end of the chapter.

Groups and group supervision

Hawkins and Shohet (2006) have identified a number of advantages of supervision in groups. First is the very issue that we identified above as contributing to the growing popularity of group supervision, that is, the economies of scale. As they point out, however, 'ideally group supervision should come from a positive choice rather than a compromise forced upon the group and supervisor' (Hawkins and Shohet, 2006). Other advantages that they discuss include opportunities for peer support and peer feedback, access to a wide range of life experiences of other members, the possibility of employing action-based techniques, and the opportunity to learn about group process and group dynamics from first-hand experience. They also highlight a number of possible disadvantages of group supervision, including being less likely to mirror the individual work which the supervisee might be conducting with patients, a preoccupation with group dynamics to the exclusion of doing any supervision, and the fact that there will inevitably be less time allocated to each individual than in one-to-one supervision.

A number of other writers have also identified general benefits of group supervision (Winship and Hardy, 1999; Clouder and Sellars, 2004; Eraut, 2004; Bulman and Schutz, 2008) and the last decade has seen a growing number of empirical research studies into the positive effects of group supervision on practice (Arvidsson, Lofgren and Fridland, 2001; Lindahl and Norberg, 2002; Linton, 2003; Enyedy et al., 2003; Lindgren et al., 2005; Jones, 2003, 2006; Alleyne and Jumaa, 2007) as well as its value in providing personal support for the practitioner (Holm, Lanz and Severinsson, 1998; Arvidsson, Lofgren and Fridland, 2001; Lindgren et al., 2005). However, it must be emphasized that group facilitation is a skilled process, and poorly-conducted group supervision can be ineffectual at best, and harmful at worst, both to the group and to the facilitator (Reichelt et al., 2009; Ogren and Jonsson, 2003).

Hawkins and Shohet make the important distinction between group and team supervision. Whereas in group supervision the group will have come together solely for that purpose, team supervision 'involves working with a group that has not come together just for the purposes of joint supervision, but have an inter-related work life outside the group' (Hawkins and Shohet, 2006). They point out that there is a crucial difference in supervision needs between teams that share work with the same clients, for example ward-based nurses, and groups of practitioners who have their own individual clients, or who share clients with other practitioners who are not in the supervision group. We will consider this in more detail later in the chapter.

Hawkins and Shohet (2006) also discuss peer supervision, that is, supervision with one or more other practitioners where no-one takes on an overt group facilitation role. Again, they highlight advantages and disadvantages, but their main concern would appear to be the danger of game-playing without realizing what is happening. Games can and do take place in most groups, but the advantage of a facilitated supervision group is that one of the jobs for which the facilitator is trained is to identify when games are occurring and to deal with them or point them out to the group members. In addition to the problem of game-playing, we would add the difficulty and possible danger which an unfacilitated group faces of not recognizing the potentially damaging impact of group dynamics.

A compromise might be to share the facilitation role between the group members, so that a different member facilitates the group at each meeting. Bond and Holland (1998) recognize this as a viable option, but point out a number of disadvantages, including a lack of authority and a lack of facilitation skills. We shall return to this issue shortly, but for now we will simply state that unfacilitated peer groups can result in a great many problems, and we would be very reluctant to recommend this model of group supervision.

While recognizing the important distinctions between facilitated groups, teams and peer groups, we have chosen to explore differences between groups in terms of function rather than structure. We have therefore distinguished between intrapersonal group supervision, interpersonal group supervision, and transpersonal group supervision.

Intrapersonal

Intrapersonal group supervision (groups which focus on the processes *within* the individual) can best be described as individual supervision with an audience. In this model, the supervisor works individually with each group member in turn while the rest of the group looks on. Clearly, it has the advantage of requiring no special facilitation skills over and above the skills of individual supervision, and, argu-ably, there is much to be learnt simply from observing the supervisory encounter, even for members who are not involved in supervision at that moment. If the intention behind establishing group supervision is purely a resource issue, then this is a model that is simple to set up and can provide supervision to an entire team of practitioners at very lit-tle financial cost. However, Bond and Holland (1998) do not recognize this as a form of group supervision, stating that 'they might as well be a queue of people waiting outside the flimsily partitioned office of a clinical supervisor, eavesdropping on what's going on'. Furthermore, they do not even view it as cost-effective, adding that 'it is a time-consuming way to provide one-to-one clinical supervision'.

Interpersonal

Interpersonal group supervision (groups which focus on what hap-pens *between* individuals) utilizes the group members as a resource. Whereas the intrapersonal group model places the supervisor clearly in the role of expert, the interpersonal model recognizes that group members also have the skills and experience to offer supervision to one another. The role of the facilitator is therefore concerned less with direct supervision than with enabling and empowering group mem-bers to supervise each other. This approach is a more efficient use of resources, and as well as receiving supervision from a number of different individuals, the group members also gain some experience of supervising others under the watchful eye of the facilitator. The interpersonal model comes closest to the definition of group supervi-sion offered by Bond and Holland (1998) of 'three or more people who come together and interrelate cooperatively with each other towards their common purpose of giving and receiving clinical supervision'. Although this is the most common model of group supervision, it views the group as nothing more than the sum of all the possible combina-tions of personal interactions, and so neglects some important aspects of group development and group dynamics.

Transpersonal

Transpersonal group supervision (groups which look *beyond* the indi-vidual) views the group as being more than simply the sum of all the inter- and intrapersonal group events. Rather, the group is seen as having a separate identity that is different from the sum of all its parts; the group, in effect, has a life of its own. We can therefore talk about 'the group' and 'group life' as if the group was a person. Indeed, some models of group development and group processes are analogous to human development from birth to death, with childhood mischiefs, adolescent identity crises and adult productivity, leading to the wisdom of old age. This model, in which the group takes on a life of its own, might account for such phenomena as group hysteria and 'lynch mobs', where the group behaves in ways that none of the individuals who comprise the group would ever dream of doing.

The group facilitator therefore has a dual role in such a group. On the one hand, she has some kind of supervisory function, either directly or indirectly, by facilitating group members to supervise each other. On the other hand, she also has a responsibility for maintaining and developing the group life, for working with 'the group' as an individual entity separate from the individuals who comprise it. Groups that follow this model are sometimes called t-groups or training groups, since one of their functions is to provide the group members with experiential learning about group dynamics. This model is particularly useful for new supervisors and group members who are interested in learning about groups by reflecting on their own practice because of its educational component. However, we would recommend that new facilitators who are planning to employ this model initially work with a skilled and experienced co-facilitator.

Reflective moment

Try to relate the above models to some of the groups of which you have been a part. These might include family groups, social groups, work-based groups and activity or recreational groups. For example, your ward hand-over might resemble an intrapersonal group in which each nurse reports on her patients in a one-to-one interaction, with other team members looking on in silence. Or it might function more like an interpersonal group in which each patient is discussed by the whole team, with everyone interacting with everyone else. Similarly, your family might resemble a loosely configured collection of individuals or it might function as a unified whole, as a transpersonal entity in its own right. You might, for example, find yourself saying things like 'my family believes in X' or responding as a family in ways that you would never do as an individual.

With a colleague, try to identify one group of each of the three types and discuss how they might function differently. For example, what would be the benefits and disadvantages if your intrapersonal ward team adopted an interpersonal model?

Group development and group dynamics

The best, perhaps the only, way to learn about group supervision is to take part in a group as either a supervisee or a facilitator. In an ideal world, you should gain experience of the former before embarking on the latter, and even then it is essential to ensure that your own practice of group facilitation is itself closely, expertly and regularly supervised by someone with experience (and preferably training) in group work. Despite the ethos of this book of learning from reflection on our practice, it is necessary to acquire some basic theory before starting. The reason for this, as we shall see, is that a great deal of what happens in groups is covert: it happens beneath the surface, it is often disguised as something else, and it is sometimes carried out unconsciously. If, as a new facilitator, you are not directed towards what to look for, you may never find it.

If we are to think of the group as a single entity, as an individual in its own right, then we need to consider how this individual develops over time. Indeed, a number of theorists have noticed that groups behave differently at different phases of their existence, and have attempted to formulate a series of stages through which groups are thought to pass. Although most of these models were constructed to explain the development of therapeutic groups, they have been widely employed with groups of all kinds.

Probably the most well-known model of group development is that devised by Tuckman (1965), who identified four stages through which a group passes, namely forming, storming, norming and performing. Tuckman noticed from a review of over 50 published papers that when groups come together for the first time, they have certain tasks to perform before they can get down to whatever business they were established to carry out. The initial *forming* stage, when the group first meets, is characterized by anxiety and a lack of direction, and the group typically looks to the facilitator for leadership. However, in many groups, the facilitator would not see such overt leadership as part of her role, and so the group is ultimately disappointed and often rebels against the facilitator. This rebellion initiates the *storming* stage, in which the role of the facilitator, and sometimes the existence of the group itself, is questioned. During this stage, group members often vie for the leadership role and the reasons for the formation of the group can be totally forgotten in the struggle for power and control. The group eventually realizes that, if any work is to be done, then the members must work together for the common good of the

group. This is the *norming* stage during which support and cooperation develops, norms and rules are established, and group members
begin to accept the facilitator's role. Finally, once all of these issues
are resolved, the group enters the *performing* stage and begins its
work.

Tuckman emphasized that not all groups pass through all four
stages (some, for example, never reach the final performing stage),
and neither do the stages always follow each other in a neat sequence.
If a group is stuck or feels threatened, for example, it might regress to
an earlier stage, just as a teenager who feels threatened might revert
to thumb sucking or acting up. He also pointed out that, although
the stages gradually follow-on from one another during the life of the
group, they are also worked through during each individual group
meeting.

Levine (1991) suggested a similar model based on sociograms,
which are pictorial representations of the patterns of communication
within the group. His *parallel, inclusion* and *mutuality* phases bear a
strong resemblance to Tuckman's stages, and are also very similar to
the stages suggested by Schutz (1958) of *in-out, top-bottom* and *near-
far* (see Table 7.1).

These models can be useful in helping us to understand how relationships between group members grow and develop during the life of
a group, and they are also invaluable for assisting the group facilitator to recognize and deal with general group dynamics such as scapegoating and subgrouping. For example, a group in its storming stage
will tend to rebel against the facilitator, perhaps even going as far as
accusing her of incompetence. By being aware of the stage at which
the group is functioning and the issues it is trying to deal with, she
can see scapegoating as a universal coping mechanism rather than as
a personal attack on her facilitation skills. Indeed, she can reframe
the attack positively as a sign that the group has progressed through
the forming stage and is developing normally, in the same way that
rebellion against parents and other authority figures is a normal sign
of personal development during the teenage years.

Reflective moment

Think back to when you joined a new group; for example, when
starting a new course or beginning a group project. Try to reflect on
the growth and development of the group, as well as its problems
and setbacks, in relation to one of the three models of group

Table 7.1 Three models of group development

Tuckman	Schutz	Levine	
Forming Characterized by anxiety and dependence on the facilitator	In-out stage Characterized by dependency on the facilitator. Group members want to be accepted and loved by her	Parallel phase Communications in the group run parallel to each other rather than across the group, and are usually directed towards the facilitator	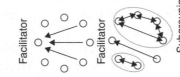
Storming Characterized by conflict, issues of leadership and rebellion against the facilitator.	Top-bottom stage Characterized by conflict and the struggle for control. The facilitator is rejected and alliances form between group members	Inclusion phase Communications towards the facilitator decrease, and those between group members increase. Fluctuating pairing and subgroupings occur. There are struggles for power and control	Subgrouping
Norming Characterized by cohesion and trust. The group begins to develop shared norms, mutual support and co-operation Performing Characterized by working on the task. The group becomes self-sufficient and functions independently of the facilitator	Near-far stage Characterized by intimacy and the formation of relationships between group members	Mutuality phase All members of the group are included. Everyone is in touch with everyone else. Empathy deepens	

development described in Table 7.1. Write a brief paragraph on each of the stages of your chosen model, focusing especially on how it felt to be in the group. For example, if you chose Tuckman's model, you might reflect on your feelings of anxiety and uncertainty during the forming phase, or on the jostling for leadership that might have occurred during the storming phase.

Although they are useful for charting the macro-dynamics of the group, these models provide only a limited picture of the minute-by-minute changes in the micro-dynamics, and offer little insight into the underlying group processes that are shaping those developments. Models such as those offered by Tuckman, Levine and Schutz provide us with a useful 'growth chart' for the group in terms of milestones that we might expect it to reach at certain points in its development; they can, as we have seen, predict childhood dependency, teenage rebellion and adult cooperation, but they provide little help in dealing with the day-to-day traumas of living with a dependent child or a rebellious teenager. For that, we need a rather more sophisticated tool.

If, as we have suggested, the analogy of the group as an individual in its own right is an accurate one, then we might expect the group to function on both a conscious and an unconscious level in the same way as a person. Furthermore, by uncovering the unconscious motivations for conscious acts, we might start to understand the day-to-day micro-dynamics of the group.

Wilfred Bion, who trained as a Freudian psychoanalyst, took just such an approach. For Bion (1989), the conscious life of the group, what he called the 'work group', is concerned with the task that it came together to carry out. In a clinical supervision group this task is, obviously, that of giving and receiving clinical supervision. However, he claimed that every group also has an unconscious life, what he called a 'basic assumption group', concerned with maintaining the group, with keeping it alive, and with responding to perceived threats to its integrity. In any group, then, what appears to be happening on the surface, the work that the group is doing, is not the whole picture. The group is also functioning on a deeper level, unbeknown to any of its individual members, according to the basic assumptions it is making about the world and the perceived threats coming both from inside and outside the group. As we have said, this 'group mentality' is held collectively by the group and is not usually present in the conscious minds of the individual group members. Furthermore, the group mentality might not correspond to the conscious mental states of *any* of the group members. For Bion, then, the group truly has a life of its own.

From Bion's (1989) experience of working with groups, he detected three basic assumptions that groups make about the perceived threats to their existence. First, there is the basic assumption of *dependency*. For Bion, one way in which the group might unconsciously deal with perceived threats is by seeking a source of security, a 'magical' person who will supply all its needs, what Bion called a group deity. The group usually turns to the facilitator to perform this function, with the assumption that when things are not running smoothly, the facilitator can make everything better. If the facilitator refuses to take on this role, the group might turn to another person, or indeed someone might nominate herself for the role, which in turn can lead to rejection or scapegoating of the facilitator. Inevitably, however, the 'group deity' will not be able to meet the expectations of the group, and will usually end up by being rejected.

The second basic assumption is *fight/flight*, in which the group unconsciously attempts to deal with its problems either by attacking them head-on or by running away from them. This is a very 'black and white' group mentality in which all other solutions apart from fight or flight are rejected. Furthermore, the welfare of individual group members is of secondary consideration. In fight mode, the problems of the group might be projected onto a particular group member, who is then scapegoated; by attacking that particular person, the group believes that it can magically destroy the problem. In flight mode, individual members might be abandoned or even expelled from the group; by ignoring the problems of a particular person, it is believed that the problems of the entire group will disappear. The paramount concern is for the survival of the group rather than of its individual members, and this scapegoating or rejection can extend to the group facilitator if she is not seen to be mobilizing the group to attack or coordinating its retreat.

The third basic assumption is *pairing*, in which the group behaves as if it will somehow 'give birth' to a saviour, who will then provide a redeeming 'big idea', through a teaming-up of two of its members. The pair can either consist of two group members or might include the facilitator, and is often interpreted by other group members as sexual in nature. Such pairings can be quite creative in the short term, but are largely unproductive since the group saviour is inevitably not forthcoming. It must be emphasized again that all of these basic assumptions are part of the *unconscious* life of the group, and the group members do not consciously and individually decide to act in a cruel or uncaring way to one another, anymore than you or I consciously decide what to dream at night.

To summaries, group supervision is sometimes employed as a more cost-effective alternative to individual supervision, but it is, in fact, something quite different and can offer far more than merely supervision with an audience. In particular, the transpersonal model regards a group as a living, thinking and growing entity that is more than, and other than, the sum of the individuals who comprise it. Not only do groups grow and develop over time, but also, like people, they need to reach a certain level of maturity before they are able to do any meaningful work. Furthermore, groups work not only on an overt conscious level, but also covertly and unconsciously, particularly when under threat. These unconscious group dynamics often manifest as individual pathologies, in which particular members (often the facilitator) are singled out for attack by the group as a whole. Left to their own devices groups can cause distress to their members and often tear themselves apart.

Further reading

Most of the classic texts on group dynamics and group process are now rather elderly, but some remain as relevant today as when they were first written. Bion (1989) is that rare thing: a source book of major importance and influence that is also very readable even for the beginner to group theory. Bion's model is nicely summarized in Wright (1989), which also deals with Tuckman, Levine and several other theorists in a concise and informative way. Wright is also one of the few writers on group work with a nursing background. For the more advanced reader, Forsyth (2010), and Yalom and Leszcz (2005) both discuss group dynamics in considerable depth.

The dangers of unfacilitated groups cannot be overstated. In this respect, you might like to think of group process and group dynamics as a useful tool for achieving specific aims, for example, as a pair of scissors. Like most tools, there are certain dangers in using it, although when used properly it can be extremely powerful. A new and inexperienced group can therefore be viewed as a young child with a pair of sharp scissors, who realizes neither the full benefits nor the dangers of what she has in her hands. Unless properly supervised, there are bound to be injuries, either to the child herself or to whoever comes near her.

Establishing the group

The remainder of this chapter is concerned with the practical issues involved in setting up and facilitating a supervision group. Like most practical skills, group facilitation can only be learnt by direct involvement in a group, and most of the reflective exercises which follow assume that you are participating in some kind of group experience, either as a facilitator or as a group member.

A number of decisions have to be taken before you start your supervision group. First, you need to decide on the basic model that your group will be following. Will it be an intrapersonal group in which you will conduct individual supervision with each group member in turn, an interpersonal group in which you will facilitate group members to supervise one another, or a transpersonal group in which your main focus will be on group process and dynamics? This is a major consideration that will influence almost every other decision you take, and so you should reflect on the three models very carefully before deciding which feels right for you.

Issues of group membership

Your next decision concerns who will be invited to join the group. This might not be your decision to take, since the membership of supervision groups is often predetermined. For example, you might be facilitating a group for a specific and well-defined clinical team in which everyone is expected to attend. However, when you do have some control over group membership, there are several well-established criteria that you should consider.

First, there is the issue of whether membership to the group should be open or closed. If your group is open, new members are able to join during the life of the group, and you might suggest or encourage members to leave before the group has run its predetermined course. Winship and Hardy (1999) point out that the constant comings and goings of an open group mirror the realities of everyday life for many practitioners and offer ways of learning to deal with the 'rivalries and micro politics of the workplace' (Eraut 2004). The advantage of a closed group (that is, one with a fixed and constant membership) is that feelings of safety and group identity are established more quickly than if members are constantly coming and going. Furthermore, the group progresses more rapidly since it does not have to backtrack when a new member joins, either deliberately to explain the group rules to the new member, or unconsciously in terms of regression to an earlier stage of development. The main disadvantage of closed groups, however, is that all groups suffer from attrition; over the life of any group, people will leave for a number of practical, personal and psychological reasons, and so it is possible that the size of the group might become economically or functionally unviable before the group has reached the end of its natural life.

This brings us to the next important consideration: that of optimum group size. Brown (1989) considered anything from three to 12 members to be the workable range for most groups, but pointed out that larger groups allow for the possibility of significantly more one-to-one relationships (three pairs in a three-person group compared to 36 in a nine-person group), a greater likelihood of sub-grouping, an increase in psychological freedom (with the increased possibility of quiet members being able to blend into the background), and more protracted problem-solving, but with better quality solutions. He went on to observe that different kinds of groups have different optimum numbers, with five to six being ideal for 'the more therapeutic person-centred type of short-term closed group' (Brown, 1989), whereas larger numbers are more appropriate for problem-solving, structured activities and open groups, where the tendency to sub-grouping can be used productively by dividing the group for certain tasks. Similarly, Nichols and Jenkinson (2006) observed that when numbers fall below six, the group usually adopts an intrapersonal model, or what they referred to as 'an observed personal counselling session'. In deciding on the number of members for your group, you should also take into account the almost inevitable dropout rate, and allow for two to three above your optimum number, especially in a closed group.

As well as deciding on the size of your group, you will also need to give some thought to its composition. First, you will need to think about whether the group is to be composed of strangers who do not have any work or social contact outside of the group, or a team of people who work and/or socialize together. In groups where members already know each other, if existing relationships are open and positive then they will usually contribute positively to the group, whereas problematic and destructive outside relationships will inevitably lead to disruptions and possibly to problems, particularly in a new group. Similarly, some members of the group might well have an outside relationship with the facilitator, and this might prove difficult where there is a power differential in that relationship, for example, if the facilitator is the boss or the assessor of one or more group members (or vice versa).

Second, there is the issue of balance within the group. This is a particularly relevant issue for multidisciplinary groups, of groups comprised of different staff grades, or of groups whose members work with widely differing types of clients, but also applies to the age, gender and culture of group members. For example, should you aim for a homogeneous group in which all members are similar in the above respects, or should you select a heterogeneous group that aims for diversity rather than conformity? As you might imagine, there is no simple answer. Homogeneity is necessary for group identity and cohesion and for what Bion referred to as the tasks of the basic assumption group (see above). However, Cleary and Freeman (2005) warned that colleagues who hold similar views may not sufficiently challenge one another, and McGill and Beaty (2001) found that this in turn could lead to a lack of progress in meeting the aims of the group. Thus, some degree of heterogeneity is important for creativity and forward movement, what Bion referred to as the tasks of the work group. This balance between homogeneity and heterogeneity is summarized in Redl's law of optimum distance, which states that groups should be 'homogeneous enough to ensure stability, and heterogeneous enough to ensure vitality' (Redl, 1951).

Expanding upon this, Bertcher (1994) argued that groups should be homogeneous on descriptive attributes such as age, gender and culture, and heterogeneous on behavioural attributes such as character type, extraversion/ introversion and leader/follower characteristics. Clearly, such decisions might be out of your control, but a good rule of thumb is to try to avoid a group in which there is one person who is too far removed from all the others on any of the above attributes. Thus, do not include someone who is much older or younger than everyone else, a lone social worker in a group of nurses, or a ward manager in a group of support workers.

Issues of time

Another important issue to be considered in establishing the group is that of time. Just as the membership of the group can be either open or closed, so too can its life-span. Open groups run indefinitely with no predetermined end point, although the life-span of open groups is often renegotiated at certain fixed intervals, such as every 20 meetings. It is possible to run a group of open life-span but closed membership, although it is likely that such a group will become smaller and smaller until it is no longer viable. It is more usual, then, for open life-span groups to have open membership (but not necessarily vice versa). Closed life-span groups can be of almost any length from six to 60 meetings, but you should be aware of allowing enough time for the group to progress through the early formative stages of development in order that there are enough remaining sessions for it to carry out its work (Platzer, Blake and Ashford, 2000; Jones, 2006). In general, short life-span groups tend to resolve issues of forming, storming and norming more quickly than longer life-span groups. For example, a six-session group might feel the urgency of time and be up and working after only two or three sessions, whereas a 20-session group might take the luxury of seven or eight sessions to resolve its forming, storming and norming issues.

The other major time issue is that of frequency and duration, of how often and how long the sessions should be. This issue might not be resolvable before the group commences, as most healthcare workers are busy people who can only spare limited time away from their work. In an ideal world, the importance of supervision will be recognized by someone in the organization with budgetary control, and provision will be made for time out from clinical work or for paid overtime to attend supervision. However, in the real world of healthcare provision, the frequency and duration of sessions is best negotiated with the group members. Generally speaking, groups should last for at least an hour, although the length of intrapersonal groups, in which each individual member is given personal supervision in turn, will depend on the number of supervisees in the group. Similarly, if your group includes interactive exercises or other structured activities, then you might find that you need at least 90 minutes, and possibly two hours for each session.

The frequency of your group is equally negotiable, but, ideally, you should aim for meetings at least fortnightly, and preferably weekly. Indeed, Saarikoski et al. (2006) considered that, for her supervision group of student nurses, weekly meetings were not frequent enough. Some groups find that they can meet only monthly, and while this might be acceptable for training or therapy groups, busy practitioners barely have a day in which issues for supervision are not raised. Some of these issues might keep for a month, but many will require far more urgent attention. If a compromise has to be made, aim for shorter but more frequent meetings rather than longer but less frequent ones.

Finally, while still on the issue of time, you should not underestimate your own time commitment as a group facilitator. As well as the one hour per week (or whatever) during which you are actually facilitating the group, you should also allow time for initial planning of the group as a whole, preparation time for each session, time to review and reflect on each session, time for writing up notes (if appropriate) and, most importantly, time for your own supervision on your role as group facilitator.

Other resource issues

We have already briefly mentioned the resources of your time as group facilitator and the time of the supervisees. Other staffing issues include a decision on the number of facilitators required (one is usual, but you might find that in a large group or where you aim to do work in sub-groups, that you need some help), issues of time and money for your own training as a group supervisor, and possible payment for an expert in group work to provide your own supervision. This is all very costly, and if you (or your organization) are considering group supervision as a cheap option to individual supervision, you should perhaps think again.

As well as staff resource issues, you also need to think about accommodation for the sessions. A quiet, well-ventilated and adequately heated room is the minimum requirement. Seating should be comfortable and, if possible, all the chairs should be of roughly the same height and design and arranged in a circle. You might also wish to provide some luxuries such as coffee-making facilities, as well as props such as flip-chart pads and pens for any written exercises and group brainstorms.

The location of the venue is also very important. For example, should the group be held in a room in the workplace where interruptions are possible, and which might have an emotional resonance for some of the supervisees, or should you opt for a less convenient but more neutral venue to which some of the group members might have to travel, and which might incur a hire cost? Connected to this is the issue of boundary protection, that is, the extent to which you are able to shut out the outside world and have a space that is truly your own for the duration of the meeting. Compromises are often necessary over the venue, but it is an extremely important issue, and you should strive for the best possible location.

Being a facilitator

Most of the research suggests that group facilitators are made rather than born. Successful group facilitation requires a combination of skills, values and attitudes that are partly acquired early in life, can partly be taught by reading or by attending courses, and are partly picked up on the job through experience. Clearly, neither this book nor any other can help you with the former; there are some skills, values and attitudes which have to be gained early in life, and if these are deficient, then you will probably never be a successful group supervisor. If, for example, you are overly domineering, do not listen to other people's points of view or are prejudiced against certain groups of people, then you should not be involved in group supervision; indeed, you should probably not be involved in healthcare at all. However, most group supervision skills and values can be learnt, and many of the caring and relationship-forming skills and attitudes that you employ as a healthcare worker are also applicable to group facilitation.

Values and attitudes

Nichols and Jenkinson (2006, p. 60) identified two important attitudes to be held by any group facilitator. First, the facilitator must value and understand the nature of personal change and growth, and second the facilitator must be open to her own feelings and those of others. They posed five questions that any prospective group facilitator should ask:

- Do you know that you are aware of and open to the flow of feelings in your daily life – do others confirm this to be so?
- Are you able to say that you value your own feelings and allow their expression rather than striving to mask them?
- Are you able to share your feelings with a trusted companion without being defensive?
- Are you able to receive and experience the feelings of others in a relaxed, accepting manner without wanting immediately to placate, soothe or distract them from expressing feeling?
- Do you judge that if a person expresses or 'acts out' feeling in a group you will be able to allow this to unfold without a panicky need to take control and return to more matter-of-fact issues?

Reflective moment

Think carefully about each of the above five questions. Reflect on your own strengths and weaknesses and write a short paragraph on each, noting where you would have something to offer a group and where you need to do some personal work. Try to identify some possible sources of help with your areas of weakness.

If you can honestly answer 'yes' to all of the above questions (and few people can!), then you probably possess Carl Rogers' three 'therapeutic conditions' of empathy, genuineness and respect, which he claimed were necessary and sufficient to bring about therapeutic change in both individual and group work (Rogers, 1961). Empathy is the sensing of the feelings being experienced by the other person, and the communication of those feelings back to her. Genuineness means being yourself, not putting up a professional front or personal façade, and expressing to the other person exactly what you are experiencing from moment to moment. Finally, respect, or what Rogers sometimes referred to as unconditional positive regard, involves communicating a positive, accepting attitude towards the other person, whatever she is expressing at the time. That is not to say that you should deny your own feelings of anger, revulsion, or whatever at what they are saying or doing, but rather that you accept and prize them as a person even though you might disapprove of their words or actions.

Facilitation skills

As well as the above attitudes, there are also a number of skills related to group facilitation. Brown (1989) suggested that these skills can be exercised in four directions, namely facilitator-group member, member-member, facilitator-group and facilitator-external environment (see Figure 7.1).

Facilitator-group member skills are employed when the facilitator needs to be able to communicate on an individual level, and are the most often used skills in the intrapersonal group model. They are also employed extensively in the first stage of group development (compare the diagram of facilitator-group member skills in Figure 7.1

Figure 7.1 Directions of group facilitation skills

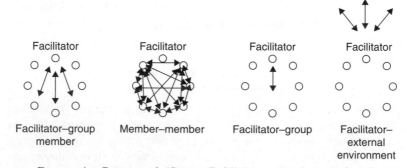

Facilitator-group member   Member-member   Facilitator-group   Facilitator-external environment

Source: Brown, A., *Groupwork* (Gower Publishing, 1992), reproduced with permission of Ashgate Publishing.

with Levine's parallel phase in Table 7.1). Member-member skills are employed to facilitate group participants to communicate with each other. They are the most often used skills in the interpersonal group model, and also correspond to Levine's mutuality phase (Table 7.1). Facilitator-group skills recognize that the group also has an identity of its own, and are the key skills in the transpersonal group model. Finally, facilitator-external environment skills acknowledge the fact that the group does not exist in a vacuum, and are utilized most often in the early stages of establishing the group, and also in the mature working stage when disclosures by group members might need to be communicated to, and negotiated with, the outside world.

Brown (1989) also distinguished between general and specific skills, where the former are the skills associated with group process (that is, with Bion's basic assumption group), and the latter are associated with the group task (that is, with Bion's work group). In our case, the skills necessary for the work group are those basic supervision skills outlined in the previous chapter, and so we will focus here on the general skills of group facilitation.

Brown identified four basic sets of general group skills, which he labelled group-creation skills, group-maintenance skills, task-achievement skills and culture-development skills. These titles are fairly self-explanatory, and correspond roughly to the skills identified by Wright (1989) of conducting, modelling, following, interpreting and analyzing, and also to Nichols and Jenkinson's (2006) three key skills for group facilitation, namely observational skills, the ability to 'take it all in'; analytic skills, making sense of what you have taken in; and work skills, keeping the group focused on their aims and goals. These skills will be explored in more detail later in the chapter.

Leadership styles

A final consideration for the facilitator of a newly-formed group is the leadership style that you intend to adopt. Much of the early research in this area identified three styles of leadership; namely, autocratic, democratic and laissez-faire. In a classic study, Lippitt and White (1953) found that democratic and autocratic leaders were both effective in task-achievement and productivity, but that a democratic style produced less dependence and resentment and greater satisfaction for group members. However, later studies suggested that the situation and function of the group are important variables, and that different leadership styles should be employed in different situations. Fiedler (1981), for example, distinguished between task leadership and group maintenance leadership, the former of which requires a more directive, cognitive and information-giving approach, whereas the latter requires a facilitative, empathic and affective approach. This model bears distinct similarities to Bion's work group and basic assumption group model discussed earlier, and suggests that the effective leader requires different skills at different points in the group's life.

Adair (2005) offered an expanded version of Fiedler's model, which included recognition of the needs of individual group members as well as group needs and task needs, and claimed that it is the leader's role to recognize these three continuously fluctuating and overlapping sets of needs and orchestrate an appropriate response. In particular, he found that a democratic style is usually preferable, but when dealing with urgent task needs, a more autocratic approach is most effective and is often appreciated by group members. Bond and Holland (1998), writing specifically about group supervision, made a similar claim that group facilitators should move gradually from short periods of being directive early on, to a predominantly 'space-giving' model of facilitation in which the group members communicate and cooperate with very little intervention from the facilitator.

We have seen, then, that there are three essential prerequisites for group facilitation. First, we need the right attitude. We should be open to and in touch with our own feelings and those of the group members, we should be honest in the expression of our feelings, and should be non-judgemental when group members express their feelings. Attitudes can be cultivated and changed, so we should not despair if we think that we do not live up to this ideal. Second, certain skills are required, including specific supervision skills and general group facilitation skills. The former were explored in the previous chapter, and the latter include the skills of maintaining and facilitating the group, of observing, interpreting and feeding back group content, and of dealing with group difficulties. All of these will be explored in more detail later in the chapter. Finally, it is necessary to be familiar with a range of leadership styles, particularly the democratic and the autocratic, and know when and how to employ them to maximum effect. These attitudes and skills cannot be attained by reading a book, and there is no real alternative to practical experience for the would-be group facilitator. As we discussed in Chapter 2, you can only gain experiential knowledge such as that required to facilitate a group by critically reflecting on the process of actually doing it.

Starting the group

There are two major tasks to be accomplished in the opening meetings of a new group: the first is to clarify the aims of the group, and the second is to agree on the ground rules.

Aims

Some groups have very broad aims, such as personal growth and development, or for members to gain insight about themselves. Supervision groups, however, usually have clearly defined task aims as well as less explicit group and individual aims. We shall start by examining the aims of the group in relation to the task for which it was convened. It is clearly not sufficient merely to dismiss the task aim as to provide supervision for the group, since the aims of supervision are themselves broad and varied, and can, for example, be directed towards providing support for the supervisee, as a means to personal, group or institutional change, as a form of education, or as an approach to problem-solving.

As facilitator, your first task is to explore exactly why the group members have joined, and what they expect to gain from group supervision. It is likely that different members will be hoping to achieve different goals, and some negotiation will probably be necessary. You should also explore openly and honestly with the group the question of whose aims it has been established to meet, which might include those of the organization, of the supervisees or of the facilitator. For example, it might be that the organization has very specific expectations for the group as a whole, which have to take priority over the aims of individual group members. There is nothing intrinsically wrong with this, as long as those aims are explicitly stated, and no attempt is made by the facilitator to impose them covertly without the knowledge of the group members. If, on the other hand, it is being left to the group to negotiate its own aims, then this should be done as democratically as possible, so that all the group members feel that they can 'sign up' to what is decided, even if it was not exactly what they anticipated. For example, some members of the group might see the aim of supervision not only to deal with work problems, but also to address personal issues if they impinge on work. However, unless all members are willing to bring personal issues to the group, resentment will quickly develop on both sides, with some members feeling that others are not contributing fully, and some feeling that others are taking up valuable group time with irrelevant personal issues.

Ground rules

If the negotiation of group aims is the first task need of the group, then establishing the ground rules is the first maintenance need. The first and most fundamental ground rule that the group will have to establish concerns confidentiality. This is a particularly important issue for supervision groups of healthcare professionals, since there is not only the problem of what any group member (including the facilitator) does with personal information that other group members might disclose about themselves, but also of what they might disclose about clients and their treatment. Both of these problems have professional as well as ethical implications. For example, what are you to do if a group member discloses that she has a criminal record for theft? Alternatively, what if she recounts an instance of unprofessional conduct? In either case you have a professional duty (and perhaps a moral duty) to discuss these revelations outside the group.

Clearly, then, in a group of this kind, confidentiality cannot be absolute. Rather, the aim of the ground rule should be to establish the limits of confidentiality and to agree on the circumstances when the facilitator (or indeed, any other group member) might communicate information to people outside the group. It is vitally important that these circumstances are made absolutely clear to every group member, since this allows them to make an informed choice about what they disclose in the group. Similarly, if it appears that someone is about to make a disclosure that might need to be communicated outside the group, then the facilitator has a responsibility to remind her of the limits to confidentiality so that she can decide whether or not to continue with her revelation.

Fortunately, big disclosures of this nature do not arise very often, and it is the smaller day-to-day issues that are usually more pressing. Most groups establish a rule that, in general, these day-to-day issues are not taken outside of the group, although the boundaries between group business and non-group business are sometimes rather fuzzy. For example, a personal issue between two group members might be brought to the group for discussion. Does it then become a group issue that can no longer be discussed outside the group by the people involved? Such a rule would clearly be debilitating, and might prevent issues being brought to the group. The usual solution to this problem is not to ban discussion of issues previously brought to the group, but to have an agreement that, when such issues are discussed, those discussions will be reported back at the next group meeting.

Apart from a rule about confidentiality, other ground rules are largely a matter of individual choice. Bond and Holland (1998) give examples of ground rules relating to autonomy and choice, to speaking for oneself, to being non-judgemental, to group commitment and to reciprocity. For some groups, these rules are largely tacit, whereas other groups prefer to state them explicitly. The problem with tacit rules is that they only become an issue when someone violates one of them and then denies that such a rule exists. For this reason, probably the most important ground rule to establish is the one that says that all rules are open to renegotiation, and that new rules can be established any time that the group feels is necessary.

Reflective moment

Most informal groups have tacit ground rules that are known to all the members but never explicitly discussed. With a colleague, think of a group of which you are both members (for example, a ward team) and try to uncover the unspoken ground rules of the group. What would be the benefits or problems of making them overt?

Running the group

In many ways, everything that we have discussed up to this point has been merely a preliminary to the real business of running the group. We have already touched on the question of what makes a good facilitator, and we shall now apply that to the broader issue of the group programme, which Brown (1989) has defined as 'what the group does as a means of trying to achieve its aims'.

The group programme

The major decision when deciding on the group programme is the degree of structure that you wish to impose. At one extreme, some groups are completely unstructured inasmuch as they are primarily 'talking groups' which focus on members discussing supervision issues with relatively little intervention from the facilitator. At the other extreme, some groups are so full of games, exercises and role plays that the structure is in danger of overwhelming the content, and there is little scope for responding to issues brought to the group by its members. A good compromise is to start the group with one or two exercises as a warm-up, and to use them as a springboard for raising supervision issues. This, of course, applies only to inter- and transpersonal models of group facilitation, since the intrapersonal model is not concerned with the group *per se*, but only with a collection of individual supervisees. However, the most important consideration is flexibility, and if someone comes to the group with a burning issue, it would be rather insensitive to press on with your pre-planned warming-up exercises, which would in any case hardly be needed.

Space does not permit a detailed discussion of the many warming-up exercises available to the group facilitator, but some suggestions of source books are given in the Guide to further reading. When planning warming-up exercises, however, it is useful to bear in mind that they serve two functions. The first is to ease group participants into the session, to loosen them up in preparation for the real work of the group. These 'ice-breaker' games might involve name-learning exercises in the forming stage of the group and trust exercises later in the storming and norming stages. Ice-breakers are often frivolous in nature, and might involve some kind of physical activity such as calling out a person's name as you throw a ball to them, or guiding a blindfolded member of the group round the room.

The second function of these exercises is to get people talking about supervisory issues, and this usually entails either a talking or writing activity such as dividing into pairs and discussing something that happened at work, or carrying out a structured reflective writing task (see Chapter 5) and sharing it with the group. As we have already mentioned, these exercises are only necessary if nothing is immediately forthcoming from the group, and even then, some facilitators prefer to work with the ensuing silence rather than deliberately breaking it with an exercise.

Once the group is working, the aim of the facilitator is largely to ensure that it continues to work. We shall discuss how the facilitator manages this process with reference to Nichols and Jenkinson's three key skills of observation, analysis and work, which we briefly mentioned earlier.

Observational skills are an important aspect of your job as facilitator, and involve not only taking in everything that is happening in the group, but also communicating your interest and attention back to the group members so that they feel valued and respected. In an intrapersonal group, your observations will focus mainly on individual group members during your interactions with them. You will be attending not only to the content of what they are saying, but to their nonverbal behaviour and paralanguage; for example, their tone of voice, their posture, their facial expression and so on. In an interpersonal group, your main focus will be on the communications between group members, with far less regard for content, which will be addressed mainly by other group members. You will be observing who is talking to whom, who the focus of discussion is, and who is excluded, and you might attempt to record these observations as sociograms (which are similar to the diagrams in Table 7.1 and Figure 7.1). Finally, in a transpersonal group, you will be observing neither individual members nor the interactions between them, but rather the 'group mood', that is, whether the group is relaxed, anxious, hostile or whatever. This requires a great deal of sensitivity and empathy, since the mood of the group is often far less tangible than the mood of its members, and might not, in fact, correspond to how any of the individuals who comprise it are feeling at the time.

Further reading

There are a number of very useful and practical books on group games and exercises. Probably the most well-known is the *Gamesters Handbook* series by Brandes and Phillips (1979), see also Brandes (1904) and Brandes and Norris (1998). These books offer a practical guide to facilitating games for social and personal development, and between them contain hundreds of games, including some specifically aimed at group leaders. In a similar vein is Bond's (1986) *Games for Social and Life Skills,* which has an excellent collection of ice-breakers, self-awareness, social skills, communication and trust games, and is a good starting point for anyone new to group games. You might also wish to explore *Effective Use of Games and Simulation* by Van Ments and Hearnden (1985), which includes games to promote change and address issues of conflict and prejudice, and *The Effective Use of Role-play,* also by Van Ments (1999), which has useful chapters on setting up and running role-play exercises, on debriefing, and on other experiential methods such as psychodrama, sociodrama and encounter groups.

Observation of what is going on in the group is not, of itself, sufficient for good facilitation, and you should also be attempting to make sense of the group behaviour. This involves the skill of analysis, and the question you should be asking yourself is: 'What is going on here?' In an intrapersonal group, your focus will be on each individual as you interact with them, and you will be offering an individual interpretation and analysis of their verbal and non-verbal behaviour. For example, you might notice that a particular individual appears anxious while she is relating what seems to be a relatively minor incident, and you will be making hypotheses about the unconscious reasons for her anxiety. In an interpersonal group, you will be attempting to understand the communications between group members, and asking yourself why certain patterns are being established, and why, for example, a usually popular group member is being ignored while a quiet member is the centre of attention. Whereas in a transpersonal group, you will be attempting to make sense of the group mood in terms of the underlying basic assumption group, and asking yourself what is going on in the group unconscious.

Through using your skills of observation and analysis, you will then be able to facilitate the work of the group, that is, the task of supervision. In an intrapersonal group, this will involve a direct supervisory input with each member in turn. A facilitator who employs this model might start with a particular person, and work around the group one by one, or else allow the group members to self-select. There is often congruence between the style in which a group is facilitated and the way in which supervision is conducted. Thus, if the supervisor chooses to facilitate the group in an intrapersonal way, then it is likely that she will conduct supervision based on the same model. For example, if a group member brings to supervision a difficulty he is having with a work colleague, the facilitator would explore the problem predominantly from the intra-psychic perspective of the supervisee by examining difficulties they have with other people in general. At times, other members might be invited to comment on specific issues, but the supervision would come predominantly from the facilitator herself. Indeed, the term 'facilitator' is not particularly descriptive of this role, and 'director' or 'leader' might be more appropriate.

In contrast, the interpersonal group facilitator, as the title suggests, is very much involved in facilitating group members to share and communicate with each other, and it is likely that this philosophy will similarly extend to her model of supervision. In the above example, then, she would not only attempt to facilitate other group members to provide the supervision, but would conceptualize the problem in terms of the interpersonal relationship between the supervisee and the work colleague. The fundamental belief underpinning this model of facilitation is that group members have the skills, experience and knowledge to offer peer supervision, and the facilitator's job is to enable that process to happen. Her direct interventions in the supervisory process will therefore be limited to helping group members when they get stuck, to correcting dangerous or obviously wrong suggestions from other group members, and to ensuring that the group sticks to its business. A successful group is one in which the facilitator says almost nothing, what Bond and Holland (1998) refer to as a 'space-giving' mode of facilitation.

The role of the transpersonal group facilitator is similar to that of the interpersonal facilitator, except that she is more likely to interpret work group issues in terms of the underlying basic assumption group, and to address them accordingly. In the earlier example of the supervisee who is having difficulties with a work colleague, the facilitator would conceptualize the issue not as a personal problem for the supervisee, nor as an interpersonal problem between the two protagonists, but as the symptom of an underlying problem in the staff team as a whole. The facilitator would therefore attempt to resolve the issue by drawing parallels between the unconscious life of the supervision group and that of the clinical team, and explore how problems in each might manifest in term of a conflict between two of the group members. The aim is therefore not to intervene directly in the business of the work group, but rather to explore the unconscious motivations for the conscious work group decisions. A summary of these three positions can be found in Table 7.2.

As pointed out earlier, a book such as this can only take you so far with your practice of group facilitation. It can provide you with what we referred to in Chapter 2 as factual 'knowing that' in the form of models and theories, and to some extent with 'knowing how' in the form of guidelines for practice, based on those models and theories. However, you will only acquire the practical experiential knowledge required by actually facilitating a group and by critically reflecting on your experience, preferably with a supervisor who is skilled and trained in group work.

Reflective moment

If you are already part of a supervision group, either as a facilitator or a supervisee, write a paragraph about how you (or your facilitator) exercise the above skills. Does your group follow one of the above models, or is it more eclectic? What are the advantages and

Table 7.2 Models of group supervision

	Intrapersonal	*Interpersonal*	*Transpersonal*
Observational skills	Observation of the verbal and non-verbal behaviour and paralanguage of individual supervisees	Observation of interpersonal patterns of communication rather than individual behaviour	Observation of the group mood and other aspects of group behaviour
Analytic skills	Individual interpretation and analysis of verbal and non-verbal behaviour	Analysis of communication patterns	Analysis of the group mood in terms of the underlying basic assumption group
Work skills	Direct personal supervision which focuses on the issues for the supervisee	Supervision by group members which focuses on the interactions between the supervisee and others in the work setting	Supervision by the group as a whole which focuses on parallels between the under-lying processes in the supervision group and those in the work team

disadvantages of a 'pure' approach to facilitation rather than an eclectic mixture of all three?

Group difficulties

It can be seen that with both the inter- and the transpersonal models the main work of the facilitator takes place when something is going wrong, and so we will now briefly consider some of the problems to which you might need to respond. Brown (1989) identified two possible causes of group difficulties. First, individual members might find themselves in problematic roles, either of their own making or because of others. Individuals take on and reject roles throughout the life of the group, and sometimes these roles are positive and facilitate the development of the group, whereas at other times they impede the group. People tend to become stuck in a role for one of two reasons. Sometimes a role is imposed on them by the group in order to fulfil a group need, for example, the role of the scapegoat, who is the repository for all of the group's problems. At other times the individual adopts a role that serves a useful short-term purpose such as avoiding a painful situation, but which is harmful or restrictive in the longer term, such as the role of 'silent member' who might have withdrawn from the life of the group when under pressure but now finds it difficult to get back in. Other typical problematic roles include the 'group patient', who can always be relied upon to bring along problems so that other group members are not forced to examine theirs; the 'group harmonizer', who smoothes over group conflicts so that difficult and painful issues are never properly dealt with; and the 'group jester', who turns difficult issues into jokes to avoid the group having to confront them.

Reflective moment

With a colleague, brainstorm some of the ways in which you might disrupt a group of which you are a member.
Your list might have included some or all of the following:

- overt or covert criticism of the facilitator or other members,
- challenging the value of the group,
- staying silent,
- dominating the group,
- intellectualizing,
- trivializing,
- scapegoating (or becoming the scapegoat),
- fidgeting, coughing, passing cigarettes or sweets,]bl[monopolizing group time, and
- seeking help but rejecting all solutions.

The second cause of group difficulties identified by Brown (1989) is when the group as a whole becomes stuck in some way. Whereas individual problems are largely symptoms of issues between group members, whole group problems are usually indicative of disputes between the group and the facilitator. For example, when your group suddenly becomes quiet, apathetic, depressed or otherwise resistant, it is probably trying to tell you something, although if Bion is to be believed, it might not consciously know just what that 'something' is. If you feel under threat from your group, you should bear in mind the following guidelines:

- Do not be defensive when criticised;
- Do not put group members down (tempting though it might be at times!);
- Do not compete with leadership challenges;
- Build on support that exists in the group; and
- Do not ignore the fact that the group is not working effectively.

The most important thing to remember, however, is not to take it personally. It is probable that the group is not unhappy with you as a person, but with your role as facilitator.

Most whole group problems, then, are concerned in one way or another with issues of authority and leadership, either with too much of it or with not enough, but whatever the problem, the solution is usually the same and involves bringing the issues into the open so that they can be discussed. Once again, the way that this is done will depend primarily on the model of group facilitation that is being employed. We will take the problem of a quiet group member as an example. In an intrapersonal group, the facilitator will address the individual with the problem, saying something such as: 'You seem to be very quiet today Andrea, I wonder if something is bothering you'. In an interpersonal group, the focus will be on the other group members and their role in initiating or perpetuating the situation, and the facilitator will say something like: 'Brian and Chris seem very talkative today, and perhaps that is preventing some of the other members from talking'. Finally, in a transpersonal group the focus will be on the group as an individual entity, and the facilitator will address her remarks to the group as a whole, saying something such as: 'I see that the group is allowing Della to remain silent today. What do you think might be the reason for this?'

Reflective moment

Think of a difficult individual that you have previously encountered in a group, either as a facilitator or a group member. Write a paragraph in response to each of the following questions:

- What effect did the difficult group member have on you; what feelings did you have; how did you respond?
- How did the difficult group member affect other group members and the task of the group?

- Did the individual get some kind of pay off for their difficult behaviour? Can you identify what it was?

___

Ending the group

Except for open life-span groups, all groups have a fixed life and a predetermined end-point. As Douglas (2000) observed, the termination of a group is part of its developmental sequence, and should therefore be anticipated and prepared for in advance. For some groups, the termination will coincide with the completion of the task for which it was established, and in these cases, the ending signals a job well done. In the case of supervision groups, however, the task must continue after the group has ended, and the termination is often seen in a more negative light, as the loss of a valuable support mechanism, almost as a bereavement. At the level of the whole group, Garland, Jones and Kolodny (1965) noted a number of typical group reactions to termination that bear a striking resemblance to the grieving process, including denial that the facilitator ever mentioned that the group was going to finish, regression to an earlier stage of development or into chaos, and rose-tinted reminiscence about the early days of the group. Similarly, at an individual level, the end of the group often triggers thoughts about other bereavements that group members have suffered in the past, including some that might not have been fully resolved at the time. The end of the group is a potentially traumatic time, and it is therefore important for it to be well-planned and presented in a positive light, as a symbol of growth rather than loss.

Nichols and Jenkinson (2006) suggested three tasks for the final session of a group:

- For the group members to reflect on the aims and outcomes of the group by discovering what each has achieved since the group started, and hence to remind themselves just how far they had come;
- To reflect on the experience of being in the group by remembering how it had been along the way; and
- To notice and share how they are now feeling at the end of the life of the group, to say their goodbyes, and to move on.

Nichols and Jenkinson went on to suggest a method of addressing these tasks that was both simple and effective:

> To assist in this task the leader was directive at this point and invited members to sit quietly for a while and try to recapture the way they had felt when first coming to the group. When they felt ready, they were to talk to one other member and listen carefully to what the other had to say, and then recount their own experience. Finally, if they wished, they could share anything they wanted to with the whole group. (Nichols and Jenkinson, 2006, p. 132)

Ultimately, though, the facilitator must put his faith in the group to say goodbye as they see fit. As Nichols and Jenkinson (2006) conclude, some groups do this in a flood of emotion, and others simply repair to the pub with very little fuss.

Further reading

There are, as far as we are aware, no books written specifically about group supervision in nursing and healthcare. However, Hawkins and Shohet (2006) devote two chapters of their text to group, team and peer-group supervision, and Bond and Holland (1998) have a very useful skills-based chapter that includes sections for both group supervisors and supervisees. In recent years, several authors have published books on therapeutic group work for practitioners in youth work, probation and community mental health nursing (Phillips, 2001), social work (Lindsay and Orton, 2008), education (Ringer, 2002) and occupational therapy (Cole, 2005), and a number of the older and more general group work texts, such as those by Brown (1989) and Douglas (2000), have a strong social work orientation that is readily transferable to nursing and healthcare.

Reflective moment

Now turn back to the aims you identified at the start of the chapter. To what extent have they been met? Write a paragraph outlining the scientific and experiential knowledge you have acquired through reading this chapter and doing the exercises. Write a second paragraph identifying any aims which you feel were only partially met or not met at all. As in previous chapters, divide your page into three columns. Head the first column 'What I need to learn', and make a list of any outstanding issues which you would like to learn more about. For example, you might wish to find out more about how to deal with difficult group members. Head the second column 'How I will learn it', and write down the ways in which your learning needs could be addressed; for example, through further reading, through attending study days, or through talking to other people. Head the third column 'How I will know that I have learnt it', and try to identify how you will know when you have met your needs.

8

Reflection-in-action

Gary Rolfe

Introduction

Most of our discussion up until now has focused on what Donald Schön referred to as reflection-*on*-action, that is, thinking about practice after and away from the scene of that practice. However, Schön also explored the concept of reflection-*in*-action, which he saw as having far more significance for professional practice, and which we see as the distinguishing feature of the more advanced practitioner. In very simple terms, reflection-in-action entails thinking about practice while doing it, and stands in contrast to reflection-on-action, in which the thought takes place after and away from the scene of the practice.

Although mindful practice of this kind might appear to be the norm, Schön noted that it is rarely recognized. Thus 'because professionalism is still mainly identified with technical expertise, reflection-in-action is not generally accepted – even by those who do it – as a legitimate form of professional knowing' (Schön, 1983). This is particularly true in nursing and the other healthcare professions, where Dartington (1994) observed that 'contemporary nursing has been dogged by a negative expectation that nurses should not think' and that 'it is an effort of will to make space for reflection in a working life dominated by necessity, tradition and obedience'. Similarly, Bond and Holland (1998) have pointed out that, although nurses are continuously making decisions and solving problems in their day-to-day practice, it is usually done at an unconscious level, and busy practitioners 'often express or display... difficulty in switching from paying attention to external events going on around to paying attention to thoughts and feelings going on within'. Particularly in nursing, the highest level of practice is usually associated with Benner's notion of the expert nurse who functions on an unconscious or intuitive level, and for whom conscious and mindful practice usually results in a deterioration in performance. However, Benner (1984) drew heavily on the work of Dreyfus and Dreyfus (1986) who recognized a similar phenomenon in most spheres of practice.

In attempting to move beyond this view of unconscious or intuitive practice, we have a number of aims for this chapter:

1. to help you to understand the complex and sometimes difficult concept of reflection-in-action as outlined by Donald Schön;
2. to discuss ways in which reflection-in-action could be applied to health and social care practice;
3. to enable you to reflect on the ways in which you might already employ reflection-in-action in your own practice; and
4. to suggest some strategies for developing your skills as a 'reflexive practitioner' through the use of reflection-in-action.

Reflective moment

Think carefully about our aims for Chapter 8. Now think about your own practice and how these aims might contribute towards developing it.

Based on our aims above, identify and write down some aims of your own, both in terms of what you hope to know and what you hope to be able to do after reading Chapter 8. We will return to these at the end of the chapter.

Reflection-in-action and the reflexive practitioner

Reflection-in-action is more than simply thinking while doing. As Schön pointed out:

> both ordinary people and professional practitioners often think about what they are doing, sometimes even while doing it. Stimulated by surprise, *they turn thought back on action and on the knowing which is implicit in action.* They may ask themselves, for example, 'What features do I notice when I recognise this thing? What are the criteria by which I make this judgement? What procedures am I enacting when I perform this skill? How am I framing the problem that I am trying to solve?' (Schön, 1983, p. 50, emphasis added).

From this description, we can see that reflection-in-action involves two separate and distinct components. First, there is the turning of thought back on action, so that unlike Benner's (1984) intuitive expert, the reflective practitioner is thinking about what she is doing as she does it. Schön (1983) also described the turning of thought back on the 'knowing which is implicit in action'. In other words, the reflective practitioner is not only conscious of what she is doing, but also of how she is doing it, of the practical knowledge that underpins her practice. Each of these components of reflection-in-action will be explored in detail, and we will conclude by suggesting some ways in which the skills of reflection-in-action can be employed and developed in health and social care practice.

Our task is made more difficult by the wealth of different terms that Schön often used to distinguish subtly different concepts, and in places we will introduce our own terminology where we feel that Schön's terms might result in confusion. However, reflection-in-action remains an elusive and difficult concept to grasp, although in our experience, practitioners who are already working at this level quickly recognize its main features.

Knowing-in-action

We shall start with the first of Schön's components of reflection-in-action, that of 'turning thought back on action'. Like many of his colleagues in the discipline of professional education, Schön was interested in the practical knowledge that accompanies skilled behaviour. For Schön, this practical 'know how' was part of the behaviour and could not be separated from it. As he pointed out, 'there is nothing strange about the idea that a kind of knowing is inherent in intelligent action' (Schön, 1983).

Further reading

Schön's notion of 'knowing-in-action' is similar to practical knowledge that we referred to in Chapter 2. Other writers, mainly from the discipline of education, have described a similar concept, and it is clearly integral to a full understanding of how practitioners think and understand the practice setting. If you wish to explore this notion of 'a kind of knowing... inherent in intelligent action' (to use Schön's phrase), you might like to look at some of these seminal texts. Usher and Bryant (1989) provide a broad overview of the issue in their chapter entitled 'Reconceptualizing Theory and Practice', while Carr

---

and Kemmis (1986) discuss the notion of theory embedded in practice in Chapter 4 of their book, and Eraut (1994) does likewise in
Chapter 3 of his. Gadamer's (1996) text offers a very readable introduction to practice theory in healthcare generally (and medicine in
particular), and Rolfe (1998), in the first two chapters of his book,
argues for a greater recognition of experiential nursing theory. More
generally, Redmond (2006) has published a useful book which looks
at all aspects of reflection-in-action across the span of social and
health care practices, and Cowan (2006) has explored reflection-in-
action for university lecturers.

This synthesis of thinking and doing, which Schön called 'knowing-
in-action', was seen as a form of practical experimentation 'which
serves to generate both a new understanding of the phenomena and
a change in the situation', such that 'when someone reflects-in-action,
he becomes a researcher in the practice context' (Schön, 1983). Thus,
if the practitioner who reflects on action is *reflective*, then the one who
reflects in action is a *reflexive* practitioner. Although Schön referred
to this level of reflexive practice as on-the-spot experimenting, he was
at pains to point out that he was not likening reflexive practice to the
controlled scientific experiment. Rather, he identified three ways in
which reflection-in-action can be seen as a form of practical experimentation or action research.

First, experimentation can be a simple pre-scientific method of
discovery through doing: as Schön put it, 'to act in order to see what
the action leads to'. This is a basic form of trial and error that Schön
described as *exploratory* experimentation, which is 'the probing, playful
activity by which we get a feel for things. It succeeds when it leads to
the discovery of something there' (Schön, 1983). Secondly, experimentation can be seen as an action that is carried out in order to produce
an *intended* change: 'any deliberate action undertaken with an end in
mind is, in this sense, an experiment' (Schön, 1983). Schön referred
to this kind of experimentation as *move-testing*. Finally, experimentation can take the form of *hypothesis testing,* which is closest to the
traditional scientific form of hypothetico-deductivism. In this mode of
experimentation, the practitioner begins with a theory about what is
happening in the practice situation, formulates an hypothesis from that
theory, and tests the hypothesis by acting on the situation. As Schön
pointed out, 'If, for a given hypothesis, its predicted consequences fit
what is observed, and the predictions derived from alternative hypotheses conflict with observation, then we can say that the first hypothesis
has been *confirmed* and the others, *disconfirmed*' (Schön, 1983).

For Schön, reflection-in-action encompasses all three modes of experimentation, such that 'When the practitioner reflects-in-action his experimenting is at once exploratory, move testing and hypothesis testing' (Schön, 1983). In healthcare practice, where actions and judgements often have to be made on the spot in a very short space of time, it is sometimes difficult to imagine how the practitioner has time to carry out even one of these modes of experimentation, let alone all three. We shall therefore begin with an example from outside healthcare, in which the practitioner has the luxury of time to think, and in which on-the-spot experimenting is done in a conscious manner.

The reflexive mechanic

Imagine, then, a car mechanic who is faced with a car that will not start. She might begin with the trial and error of *exploratory* experimenting, in which she simply tinkers with various wires and components. At this point, she has no clear ideas about why the car will not start, and is merely speculatively probing with no real expectation that it will resolve the problem. She might be lucky and find that the problem was caused by a loose wire that she has inadvertently moved back into place, but otherwise she will have to progress to the next stage of *move-testing*. In this case, the moves are deliberate and are intended to produce a particular outcome. The mechanic might test out the possibility that the spark plugs are damp by replacing them with a fresh set, or that the fuel pipe is blocked by looking to see whether any petrol is reaching the carburettor.

This approach works very well for simple problems, but most situations that mechanics and healthcare practitioners have to deal with are far more complex. The mechanic might narrow down the problem to the fact that there is no spark at the plugs. Now, there are many reasons why this might occur: a flat battery, damaged leads or faulty plugs, to name but three. Of course, there are many reasons for each of these three causes. A flat battery might be caused by physical damage to the battery itself, by dirty connections, or by a broken alternator. As we can see, a simple move testing approach to resolving the problem might take some time, and if the problem is caused by two or more faults, then a linear approach in which potential causes are tested one by one might never uncover the problem.

This, then, brings us to Schön's third form of experimenting, that of *hypothesis-testing*. The aim here is not merely to try out simple moves such as replacing the spark plugs, but to formulate theories from the given symptoms. Our mechanic might have observed that there is no spark at the plug, but that the move testing strategy of replacing the battery only temporarily rectified the problem. She might theorize from this that the alternator is broken, which in turn is shorting out the battery and causing it to discharge. This theory would generate the hypothesis that the problem would be resolved by replacing the battery *and* the alternator at the same time. The hypothesis could then be tested by doing just that, and if the car now starts, then the hypothesis is confirmed (or, at least, strongly supported) and the mechanic has both generated knowledge about the car and fixed it by the same action. Clearly, such hypothesis-testing approach requires a deep understanding of the situation that encompasses both scientific and experiential knowledge.

Reflective moment

Recall a situation from your practice in which you have had to make an on-the-spot judgement or assessment. With a colleague, discuss how you came to your clinical decision. Did you follow any of Schön's three forms of experimenting? If not, can you identify any sort of rational process, or were you acting 'intuitively'?

The reflexive healthcare practitioner

It might be argued that this model is all very well for car mechanics who are able to stop and think at every stage of fixing the car, but that there simply is not enough time in the midst of practice for the health-care practitioner to employ this kind of reasoning to her on-the-spot clinical decisions. This was the view expressed by Benner (1984) in her book *From Novice to Expert*, where she provided a number of examples of nurses who intuitively knew the right thing to do without having to think about it. For example, she cited a mental health nurse who claimed:

> When I say to a doctor, 'the patient is psychotic', I don't always know how to legitimize that statement. But I am never wrong. Because I know psychosis from inside out. And I feel that, and I know it, and I trust it. I don't care if nothing else is happening, I still really know that. (Benner 1984, p. 32)

Benner claimed that the nurse was unable to legitimize her statement because her practice knowledge was not the result of a rational process; the nurse could not think about the reason for her observation because there was, in effect, nothing to think about. However, Schön disagreed with this view and suggested that the thought and the action components of reflection-in-action are actually two parts of the same process, what he described as 'a continual interweaving of thinking and doing'. The thinking component is a form of *practical* thinking, of thinking through doing, while the doing component is a *thoughtful* doing. Thus, the practitioner

> does not separate thinking from doing, ratiocinating his way to a decision that he must later convert to action. Because his experimenting is a kind of action, implementation is built into his inquiry. (Schön, 1983, p. 68)

Furthermore, for Schön, this process usually occurs so rapidly that it is performed unconsciously; what the baseball players whom he studied referred to as 'finding the groove', and what the jazz musicians spoke of as 'getting a feel for the music'. This might be the reason why some practitioners refer to their on-the-spot decisions as intuitive. However, he also argued that practitioners are sometimes able to construct a 'virtual world' in which the pace of action can be slowed down in the practitioner's head so that *conscious* reflection is possible. Thus:

> Even when the action-present is brief, performers can sometimes train themselves to think about their action. In the split-second exchanges of a game of tennis, a skilled player learns to give himself a moment to plan the next shot. His game is the better for this momentary hesitation, so long as he gauges the time available for reflection correctly and integrates his reflection into the smooth flow of action. (Schön, 1983, p. 279)

The first aspect of reflection-in-action, then, is the conscious and mindful attention to the task at hand. The healthcare practitioner is sometimes able to stop and think in the midst of action and to describe and articulate the situation as they see it; unlike Benner's example of the 'intuitive' mental health nurse, they are able to give a report of *why* the patient is psychotic rather than 'just knowing it'.

This conscious articulation of the situation is important, particularly when the practitioner is called upon to justify actions or to teach them to others. However, as we have seen, there is a second aspect to reflection-in-action in addition to simply being mindful. As Schön noted, not only is the reflexive practitioner aware of her thoughts as she practices, but '[s]he also reflects from time to time on [her] own performance, asking, in effect, Just what is it I spontaneously do in this situation?' (Schön, 1987). Bond and Holland (1998) described this

Figure 8.1 Three levels of reflection-in-action

Healthcare intervention	➡	'Intuitive' doing
Reflection on the intervention	➡	Thinking about doing
Meta-reflection on the reflection	➡	Thinking about thinking about doing

as 'Level 4' reflection, in which the practitioner is not only aware of her own thought processes, but is also aware of her awareness of those thoughts. They borrowed Casement's (1985) term 'internal supervisor', since the practitioner is, in effect, acting as her own supervisor as she practices. We shall use the term 'meta-reflection' for this process of reflecting on our own reflections. Reflection-in-action therefore involves doing, thinking about doing, and thinking about thinking about doing (Figure 8.1).

The main difference between Benner's intuitive expert and the reflexive practitioner, then, is that the latter is aware of her *modus operandi*, her methods of practice. Furthermore, she is not only reflecting on the details of the situation she is dealing with, but is also meta-reflecting on the process of how she is dealing with the situation.

Reflective moment

Return to your reflective writing about your on-the-spot clinical judgement. At which of the three levels described in Figure 8.1 were you working? Write a paragraph to explore your reflection-in-action in this case.

Towards a model of reflexive practice

We can see, then, that reflection-in-action is far more than simply thinking about practice while doing it. First, it involves a form of on-the-spot experimenting which brings together thinking and doing in a single act, and which Schön sometimes referred to as 'knowing in action'. Second, it also involves a meta-reflection on the process of knowing in action as it is taking place (see Figure 8.2).

However, we saw earlier that Schön also divided the process of knowing in action or on-the-spot experimenting into three types,

Figure 8.2 A basic model of reflection-in-action

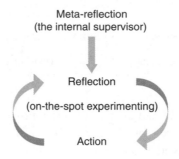

namely exploratory, move-testing and hypothesis-testing. In order to explore these further, we have associated each type of experimentation with a particular mode of thinking, doing and knowing (Table 8.1).

This, of course, is an enormously over-simplified model of a very complex process, which we have constructed merely to facilitate thinking about reflection-in-action. In other words, the aim of the model is to stimulate your 'internal supervisor' rather than to provide a definitive description of how it functions.

Table 8.1 A model of knowing in action

	Thinking	*Doing*	*Knowing*
Exploratory experimentation	Engaging with the problem	Pre-theoretical probing (trial & error)	General knowledge and theory
Move-testing experimentation	Understanding the problem	Knowledge-based action	
Hypothesis-testing experimentation	Theorizing/ hypothesizing about the problem	Theory-based action	Specific knowledge and 'theory of the unique case'

The reflexive practitioner

We will now use Benner's expert mental health nurse as an example of how a healthcare practitioner might reflect-in-action. You will recall that Benner's nurse always knew when a patient was psychotic, even though she could not always say how she knew. Benner's explanation was that the nurse was engaged in some form of unconscious and arational pattern-matching that could not be explained in words. However, it is also possible to account for her expertise in terms of Schön's notion of reflection-in-action. When she first meets the patient, the nurse has very little specific knowledge about him, and must rely on her broad knowledge of psychiatric patients in general. In her attempt to engage with the problem, her reflections are exploratory and her actions are based largely on trial and error, and correspond roughly to the car mechanic's initial tinkering (see Table 8.1 above). At this point she will have a number of possible diagnoses and treatment plans in her head, with little to guide her decisions about which might be the correct one.

As she gets to know the patient (which, for a skilled mental health nurse, might happen very quickly), she switches into move-testing mode (see Table 8.1). Her questions to herself now become more focused: 'Is this person depressed?'; 'What is the cause of his depression?'; Are his fears real or delusory?'. She might ask questions of the patient to test her growing understanding of the problem: 'How long have you felt this way?'; 'Do you feel worse at night or in the morning?'; 'Does anything help to relieve your depression?'. Her actions are no longer based solely on trial and error, but arise from her growing knowledge and understanding of the patient and his condition, as well as from established theories about psychosis and depression. She continues to reflect on the problem, but her thoughts now have more shape and direction.

As the nurse continues to build upon her understanding of the patient, she begins to develop her own personal theory about the presenting problem, what Schön called her 'theory of the unique case'. Perhaps his depression was caused by a loss; perhaps it is the depressive phase of a bipolar disorder; perhaps it is part of a toxic confusional state. At this point, her interventions will be centred around testing hypotheses based on these theories. If, for example, she theorizes that the depression is symptomatic of a toxic state, then she will ask questions about fluid intake and might suggest blood tests to confirm or disprove her hypothesis. Her actions are therefore determined by her thoughts and theories, and those theories are in turn confirmed or modified by the results of her actions. This reflexivity of thinking and doing is precisely what Schön meant when he wrote about the on-the-spot experimenting that is so characteristic of reflection-in-action.

However, as we have seen, this on-the-spot experimenting or knowing in action is only part of the story of reflection-in-action, which also includes a meta-reflection on the process. Thus, not only is the practitioner reflecting on the *content* of the practice situation ('if this patient is suffering from an acute toxic state, there is likely to be a spontaneous remission over the next 48 hours'), but she is also reflecting on the *process* of her reflective thoughts ('I am setting up an hypothesis which will confirm or disconfirm my theory'). The reflexive practitioner is therefore aware not only of the thoughts and reflections that underpin her judgements and decisions, but also of the ways by which she arrives at those thoughts and reflections. This meta-reflection is important if the practitioner is to explain and teach her skills to colleagues rather than merely to demonstrate them.

Reflective moment

Write a brief description of a practice decision that you made intuitively. Attempt to reconstruct what you were thinking as you formulated your decision. To what extent were you aware of those thoughts at the time? Now write a paragraph in which you meta-reflect on those thoughts by asking yourself Schön's question: 'Just what is it I spontaneously do in this situation?'

As we emphasized earlier, this model is a gross oversimplification of the way in which the reflexive practitioner arrives at her clinical judgements. In particular, it is unlikely that she will work sequentially through the three stages to arrive at a neat solution. She might, for example, begin with a hypothesis and only revert to the trial and error stage of exploratory reflection-in-action if her hypothesis is disproved. However, the important point that we wish to make is not about the exact nature of the process, but rather that such a process is possible. Contrary to Benner's view, we are claiming that healthcare practitioners can not only reflect and meta-reflect on their practice while they are practicing, but more importantly that this reflection-in-action can help them and their colleagues to be better practitioners.

The reflexive practicum

Having explored Schön's notion of reflection-in-action, we will now turn our attention to his concept of the practicum as the means of developing the reflective skills of the advanced practitioner. Schön defined a practicum as:

> a virtual world, relatively free of the pressures, distractions, and risks of the real one, to which, nevertheless, it refers. It stands in an intermediate space between the practice world, the 'lay' world of ordinary life, and the esoteric world of the academy. (Schön, 1987, p. 37)

Sometimes the practicum is located in a classroom, sometimes it is located in a laboratory, and sometimes it is part of the real-life practice setting. However, a practicum is more than simply a physical space, since 'it embodies particular ways of seeing, thinking and doing that tend, over time, as far as the student is concerned, to assert themselves with increasing authority' (Schön, 1987). A practicum therefore also includes a theory of professional practice. In fact, Schön identified three types of practicum, related to different kinds of professional knowledge. First, there is the technical practicum which aims to train the student in the 'correct' ways of solving problems for that particular profession by teaching her the facts, rules and procedures that members of the profession generally apply. In the second kind of practicum, the student is taught not only the facts and rules, but also the practical strategies that the professionals use to apply those rules. This kind of practicum operates at a deeper level, but it still teaches the student that there is a right response to every situation.

In healthcare education, we can see these two kinds of practicum in the classroom and the skills laboratory. First, the student is taught the facts, and second she is taught how to apply them. However, it is only when the student is in the actual practice setting with actual practitioners and clients that the third kind of practicum is encountered. This 'reflective practicum' acknowledges 'neither that existing professional knowledge fits every case nor that every problem has a right answer', and focuses on 'the reflection-in-action by which, on occasion,

Table 8.2 Schön's three types of practicum

	Usual location	Focus	Coach
Technical practicum	Classroom	Teaching the facts	Teacher
Applied practicum	Laboratory	Applying the facts	Teacher or practitioner
Reflective practicum	Practice setting	Dealing with unusual situations	Practitioner

students must develop new rules and methods of their own' (Schön, 1987). These three types of practicum are summarized in Table 8.2.

Reflective practicums are largely outside the control of the academy, and 'depend for their effectiveness on a reciprocally reflective dialogue of coach and student' (Schön, 1987). The role of the coach is rather different from that of the supervisor that we discussed in Chapter 6, since the supervisor tends to facilitate reflection-on-action outside the practice setting, whereas the coach will be working alongside the student in the clinical arena. In healthcare, we often refer to the coach as a mentor, whose role has been described in nursing as 'sharing their experience, thus teaching the best way of doing things, enhancing their proteges' skills and furthering their intellectual ability' (Butterworth and Faugier, 1998). However, Butterworth and Faugier continue by noting that 'such a demanding role obviously requires a competence over and above that of simply being able to function as a trained nurse'. In particular, many of the practitioners who will be fulfilling the role of mentor will not be skilled in initiating the kind of reflective dialogue demanded by Schön. Like Benner's mental health nurse, their ability to articulate the inner processes of their clinical decision-making will often be severely limited. If we are to facilitate the first generation of practitioners to reflect-in-action, then we cannot rely on the hit-and-miss environment of the 'raw' clinical area for our practicum.

Further reading

You might wish at this point to read a little more widely on the role of the mentor. This role is discussed by Butterworth and Faugier (1998) in chapter 1 of their book, where they contrast it with clinical supervision; it is given extensive treatment in chapter 2 of Morton-Cooper and Palmer (2000); and is briefly discussed in chapter 1 of Bond and Holland (1998). A more recent discussion of mentorship specifically in relation to reflective practice can be found in chapter 4 of Bulman and Schutz (2008). You might also wish to consider the extent to which these roles differ from Schön's description of the reflexive coach.

The practice area is not the ideal location for a reflective practicum, not only for practical reasons, but also for emotional ones. As Schön observed:

For the student, having to plunge into doing – without knowing, in essential ways, what one needs to learn – provokes feelings of loss. Except in rare cases, students experience a loss of control, competence, and confidence; and with these losses come feelings of vulnerability and enforced dependency. It is easy, under these circumstances, to become defensive. (Schön, 1987, p. 166)

Similarly, the coach or mentor

must accept the fact that he cannot tell his students about [practice] in any way they can at first understand, and then he must cope with their reactions to the predicament in which he has helped to place them. (Schön, 1987, p. 166)

In the healthcare professions, not only must the student and mentor deal with feelings of inadequacy at not being able to master the tasks at hand, but also with feelings of anxiety. Unlike Schön's examples of the architect and the musician, the healthcare practitioner is working with vulnerable people, often in life or death situations, and therefore does not have the luxury of 'doing without knowing' or learning from her mistakes. What is required, then, is a *reflexive* practicum, a 'virtual messy world' in which the student can experiment with alternative approaches to problems for which the accepted solutions do not work, and in which the action can be slowed down or stopped altogether in order to allow her to explore her own reflection-in-action.

Live supervision as a practicum

We wish to suggest one such approach to constructing a reflexive practicum that originated in the practice of family therapy. This approach is called live supervision, and, as its name suggests, it involves supervision *during the therapeutic encounter* from one or more colleagues. Live supervision was devised by Braulio Montalvo (1973) as a training technique for novice family therapists, and was later extended to team work with peers (Brown, 1984), where it is sometimes referred to as live consultancy. Clearly, however, it has potential benefits in situations other than family therapy.

The main advantage of having access to clinical supervision during practice rather than afterwards is that it can address both the ongoing and developing situation and also the process by which the practitioner is responding to that situation (her meta-reflection). Furthermore, it is far more reflexive than traditional supervision, since suggestions can be immediately implemented without having to wait until the next meeting. Live supervision therefore provides training in the advanced skill of reflection-in-action for practitioners at all levels from student to expert, and integrates the traditional roles of clinical supervisor and mentor.

Unlike many healthcare interventions, live supervision involves a team, typically with two to four members (Reimers and Treacher, 1995). One team member (whom we will refer to as the therapist) will be actively involved with the patient, while the other team members (the supervisors) will observe and occasionally intervene. There are a number of possible interventions that the supervisors could make. They might offer their own *hypotheses* about the ongoing therapeutic process, their *interpretation* of the interactions between the therapist and the patient, or simply provide *feedback* and *directions* to the therapist. As well as these more or less direct interventions, they might also offer *time out* from a difficult session for the therapist to collect her own thoughts. A discussion of the full range of possible interventions is provided by Kingston and Smith (1983).

The reflexive practicum for live supervision straddles the worlds of practice and education, and although it is most appropriately situated in a clinical setting, that setting requires some modification. The simplest arrangement is for the team of supervisors to be present in the room in which the therapist is practicing (Kingston and Smith, 1983). However, this is not always an ideal situation, and it is often preferable for the supervisors to be physically separated and to view the session through a one-way mirror or on a video screen. This arrangement provides a number of options for live supervision. The most usual intervention involves the supervisors calling the therapist out of the room to offer one or more of the above forms of intervention. On other occasions, the therapist might recognize that she is stuck and leave the room to consult with her supervisors, while in exceptional cases, the supervisors might enter the room and directly intervene in the therapeutic process.

As you might expect from such an unusual approach to supervision, there are a number of difficulties. First, there is the problem of extending an approach that was devised specifically for the practice of family therapy to the wider arena of health and social care practice, and it is important to recognize that there are certain settings in which it is not appropriate to employ live supervision. Second, live supervision runs counter to the expectations of clients, who are generally not used to having their treatment observed, nor to having their therapist called away at intervals during their treatment. Third, it is undeniably resource-intensive, particularly in terms of staff.

However, there are also a number of very valuable benefits to be had from live supervision. We have already seen how the supervisors can help the therapist in formulating hypotheses and generally making sense of the therapeutic situation, and can offer time out for the therapist to reflect and regain her thoughts. In addition, live supervision can offer added support and safety to both the therapist and client, and can help to prevent burnout (Burnham, 1986). It is an ideal training tool for students and junior practitioners, and can increase flexibility and innovation in more senior staff by bringing fresh pairs of eyes and new perspectives to their practice.

We will now explore some of the ways in which live supervision can be utilized in practice. We shall begin with an example from family therapy, and then discuss how it can be applied to a wide range of more common forms of health and social care practice. This is an actual case that one of us encountered when working in a family therapy team, which we shall discuss with reference to the model of knowing in action presented in Table 8.1.

Case example: The bereaved father

Mr and Mrs Adams, both of who were thirty years old, had been referred for Mr Adams' unresolved grief following the death of their six-month-old son two years previously. The child was Mr Adams' first, although his wife had two daughters from a previous marriage. In the initial interview, the team learned that the baby died in his sleep during the night, and was discovered by the husband the following morning, who attempted to resuscitate him without success. Mr Adams claimed to feel particularly to blame since his wife had been out the previous evening and he had put the child to bed. When asked how he was now, he replied that he felt 'numb'. At this stage, the therapist hypothesized that, as well as feeling guilty and responsible for the death, Mr Adams might be feeling angry with his wife for being out and with the other children for being alive whilst his biological child was dead, and that these feelings of anger had been repressed, leading to him becoming stuck in the grieving process. We can see that, in this case, the therapist moved immediately to the hypothesis-testing mode of experimentation with a fully-formulated hypothesis.

The supervisory team of two trained family therapists and a student, who were observing through a one-way mirror, were less certain of this straightforward interpretation. However, they had no clear hypothesis of their own at this stage, and therefore reverted to the exploratory mode of experimentation. They did this by calling the therapist out and giving her the instruction to ask Mr Adams to talk about his feelings in the week following the death. She returned to the room and did so, and at this point Mr Adams became very angry and listed a catalogue of issues which he felt had been dealt with very badly by the hospital. These included a post-mortem being carried out against his will, seeing his son in the hospital chapel with the incisions from the post-mortem on full display, and being persuaded by the chaplain not to pursue his wish for the child to be buried in his garden.

This pre-theoretical probing produced some new information that allowed the therapist to see that Mr Adams' anger was not being repressed, but was simmering just below the surface. The therapist therefore refined the hypothesis to one of displaced anger, and left the room to consult with the supervisory team. Her question at this point was 'how is this man dealing with his anger?', and the supervisors suggested some move-testing experimentation to explore how Mr Adams was working through his feelings. He was initially very reluctant to discuss this issue, but it eventually emerged that he had coped with his distress by drinking 12 to 15 pints of beer every night and keeping a drunken vigil at the grave-side in the local cemetery in the early hours of the morning. His job was at risk because he was not sleeping, and his marriage was in crisis.

At this point, the supervision team further refined their hypothesis: Mr Adams was experiencing anger at a range of people (including himself) whom he could not confront either because they were inaccessible (the hospital staff) or because it seemed inappropriate (his wife and children). Seen in this light, his drinking was an unconscious attempt to punish himself and his family, and at this point the therapist left the room for a third time to discuss ways of testing this hypothesis and of helping the man to acknowledge and begin to address the problem.

The team decided to confront the problem head-on by employing the 'empty-chair' technique. First, the wife was asked to imagine her husband in an empty chair that was facing her, and to tell him how she really felt about his drinking. This technique enabled her to say things to him that she could not say to his face, and she spoke for some time about her sadness at losing not only her child, but also her husband. Then it was her husband's turn. He was initially very resistive, but slowly began to tell his wife, through the empty chair, how he blamed her for not being there to put their son to bed, and how he was angry that she appeared to have come to terms with the death; indeed, to have almost forgotten about their son. The session ended with tears and some contemplative silences. This empty-chair work therefore not only confirmed the team's hypothesis, but also began to address the problem.

Figure 8.3 A map of a session

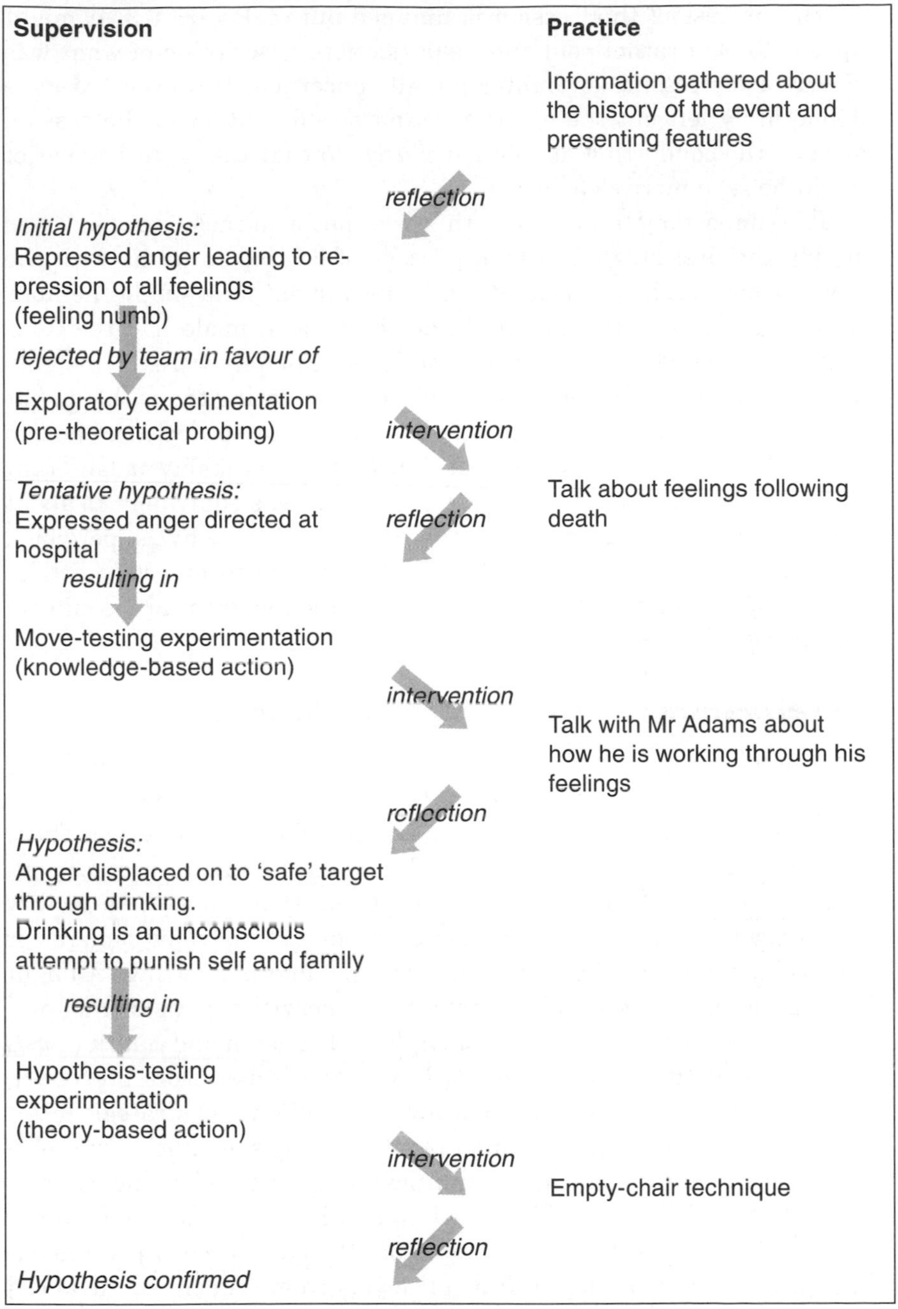

Supervision	Practice
	Information gathered about the history of the event and presenting features

reflection

Supervision	Practice
Initial hypothesis: Repressed anger leading to re-pression of all feelings (feeling numb) *rejected by team in favour of* Exploratory experimentation (pre-theoretical probing)	

intervention

| *Tentative hypothesis:*
Expressed anger directed at hospital | Talk about feelings following death |

reflection

resulting in

Move-testing experimentation (knowledge-based action)

intervention

Talk with Mr Adams about how he is working through his feelings

reflection

Hypothesis:
Anger displaced on to 'safe' target through drinking.
Drinking is an unconscious attempt to punish self and family

resulting in

Hypothesis-testing experimentation (theory-based action)

intervention

Empty-chair technique

reflection

Hypothesis confirmed

The process of this session is mapped out in Figure 8.3. It might appear to be a rather cold and dispassionate description of what was clearly a distressing encounter for all concerned. However, we have deliberately left out the emotional and social content of the session such as the comforting and empathizing, so that the cognitive aspect might be seen more clearly.

It is important to note that this was not a miracle cure, but was simply the first stage in a long process of coming to terms with the death. However, it was a significant achievement for a single one-hour session, and such progress would not have been made had the technique of live supervision not been employed. Not only were the insights and hypotheses of the team essential for formulating the problem, but the possibility for the therapist to take time out towards the end to think about how to move the session forward probably meant that the progress which the team made in an hour was equivalent to about three sessions of traditional therapy. In addition, the live supervision had enabled the therapist to develop her ability to reflect in action, and had provided the student with a valuable insight into the clinical reasoning of a skilled practitioner.

Establishing a reflexive practicum

Although the reflexive practicum of live supervision was developed by family therapists, it can be applied far more widely to almost any setting in which non-routine practice is (or should be) taking place. There are, of course, a number of issues that must be taken into account, but most can be resolved quite easily. First, there must be a facility for observation. In some settings, equipment such as video cameras or one-way mirrors could be installed, whereas in other settings it might be more appropriate simply to have the supervision team sitting quietly and unobtrusively in a corner. Indeed, Kingston and Smith (1983) pointed out that one advantage of having the supervisors present in the room is that it introduces another powerful form of strategic intervention in which the supervisors are 'apparently speaking to the therapist but intending that the communication is received by the [client]'. Second, the team must decide in advance who will be acting as therapist and who will be offering supervision. We have already pointed out that it is appropriate for staff at all levels from student to advanced practitioner to take on any of the roles. For example, a team might consist of a qualified practitioner acting as therapist, with other practitioners and students as supervisors. This arrangement provides the practitioner with important feedback on her performance and gives the more junior staff an opportunity to observe and discuss high-level practice. Alternatively, the student might be acting as therapist, in which case she is able to receive expert guidance and evaluation from advanced practitioners.

Third, it is vital that the patient is aware of this rather unusual method of working and gives her full and informed consent. It might be useful to point out to the client that live supervision is a training tool which will maximize safety and best practice, and that it is the therapist who is being observed rather than the client. However, it can still be a daunting prospect for the client, particularly when the practice intervention is painful or intimate. It is sometimes better in such cases for the supervisors to be present in the treatment room rather than to monitor the situation with a video camera, since the client can never be certain of just who is watching the video monitor, or indeed whether a recording is being made. In any case, it is important that the client is introduced to the whole team before the therapeutic intervention, is reassured about confidentiality, and is given the opportunity to ask questions about such an unusual working arrangement.

Finally, we noted earlier that live supervision is most appropriate in non-routine situations where the therapist is called upon to make professional judgements about problems that are not found in the text books. There might be some small advantage to giving live supervision to a nurse while she is making a bed, but it will be far outweighed by the cost implications.

Reflective moment

Think about your own practice setting and discuss with a colleague from a similar setting how you might establish a live supervision practicum. In particular, think about who you might include in the team, how you would monitor practice, and some of the obstacles that you would need to overcome

The reflexive practicum in action

We shall now briefly discuss a number of health and social care settings in which the reflexive practicum of live supervision might be appropriate. As we have already noted, live supervision is of most value in situations where non-routine decisions and professional judgements have to be made in a well-controlled setting, particularly where the action can be slowed down or stopped altogether as and when required. One obvious situation in which live supervision could be of great benefit is the admission or assessment interview, particularly if it is seen as an opportunity to understand the client and make a diagnosis of care rather than merely as a form-filling exercise. The simplest and least threatening arrangement of the assessment interview as a reflexive practicum is for a single supervisor to be present in the room while the assessment is conducted. The supervisor is then able to make hypotheses and judgements about care options and can intervene directly or call the assessor out of the session to offer feedback and suggestions. Furthermore, the arrangement works equally well with the more experienced practitioner as either therapist or supervisor, and provides a mutual learning experience for both practitioners.

A similar but more specialized setting is the practice nurse's surgery, since almost every new clinical encounter will involve some degree of assessment. As above, the most appropriate setting is for the supervisor to be present in the room and to intervene as required. This arrangement is an ideal training environment for the novice practice nurse, since it enables her both to observe a more experienced colleague in action and to practice under the watchful eye of an expert supervisor.

There are also a number of situations that are more conducive to a team of supervisors situated outside of the immediate practice area. An obvious example would be in group work, where a multidisciplinary supervision team might view a social skills group run by an occupational therapist or social worker through a one-way mirror. This setting would be very similar to the family therapy example described above, in which the team would call out the therapist at regular intervals to offer hypotheses and feedback, and provides an ideal environment for trainee group facilitators to observe and participate in group work. It could also, of course, be used as a way of conducting group supervision as described in Chapter 7.

Finally, and more radically, it might be possible to install a video camera in a minor-injuries cubicle in an Accident and Emergency department of a hospital. It would, of course, be necessary to obtain consent from all patients who were treated in this 'live' cubicle, but it would provide an extremely effective multidisciplinary training facility which would enable junior staff from all professions to learn from their more senior colleagues.

These are just four of many different ways in which live supervision could be incorporated into everyday practice. As we have seen, it is an expensive and often challenging approach to practice, but it offers an unusual and very effective method for practitioners from all disciplines and at all levels to develop the ability to reflect in action which Donald Schön and other writers see as essential for advanced practice. Furthermore, it offers an opportunity for students, novice practitioners and experts to explore the underlying thought processes of practice (what Schön called 'knowing in action') that often go unnoticed in the pressures of their everyday work.

Further reading

If you are planning to incorporate live supervision into your practice, we recommend that you read about how it has been employed in family therapy. Many of the key works such as Montalvo (1973) and Kingston and Smith (1983) were published some years ago in specialist journals that might be difficult to obtain, and so you might find it easier to read some of the many summaries that have appeared in textbooks. A good place to start is with John Carpenter's chapter 'Working Together: Supervision, Consultancy and Coworking' in Treacher and Carpenter (1992). Philip Barker's (2007) book includes a useful chapter entitled 'Teaching and Learning Family Therapy', which explores a number of training methods including live supervision, and Reimers and Treacher (1995) also discuss live supervision with and without a one-way mirror in their chapter entitled 'Research and Practice, Practice and Research'. To the best of our knowledge, there are no nursing or general healthcare texts that explore the use of live supervision.

Reflective moment

Now turn back to the aims you identified at the start of the chapter. To what extent have they been met? Write a paragraph outlining the learning about reflection-in-action you have acquired through reading this chapter and doing the exercises. Write a second paragraph identifying any aims which you feel were only partially met or not met at all. As in previous chapters, divide your page into three columns. Head the first column 'What I need to learn', and make a list of any outstanding issues which you would like to learn more about. For example, you might wish to find out more about live supervision. Head the second column 'How I will learn it', and write down the ways in which your learning needs could be addressed, for example, through further reading, through attending study days, or through talking to other people. Head the third column 'How I will know that I have learnt it', and try to identify how you will know when you have met your needs.

9

Using reflection as a tool for research

Dawn Freshwater

Introduction

In this chapter the relationship between reflection and research is examined and situated within the debate initiated in Chapter 2 around evidence based practice, paradigms and paradigm shifts and the search for truth. Research approaches that specifically use reflection are explored in order to illustrate ways of finding and validating knowledge in healthcare settings. Such approaches include storytelling and narrative, action research, feminist research and various other so-called 'postmodern' approaches. Until now, we have discussed the concepts of reflection and critical reflection as ways of improving practice through writing, individual and group supervision and critical thinking. We now turn to reflection and reflexivity as tools for improving practice through research.

Our aims for this chapter are:

1. To explore the relationship between reflection and research;
2. To outline the difference between reflection, critical reflection and reflexivity as approaches to research;
3. To explore the relationship between reflexivity and evidence based practice; and
4. To explore the role of the researcher in reflexive research.

Reflective moment

Having looked at our aims for this chapter, take some time to consider what you understand the relationship between research and reflective practice to be. Some questions to ponder might include: How might reflection be used to add value to the research process? How could reflecting on clinical practice be understood as a form of inquiry?

Based on our aims above, identify and write down some aims of your own, both in terms of what you hope to know and what you hope to be able to do after reading Chapter 9. We will return to these at the end of the chapter.

Research and reflexivity

Reflexivity is a frequently used term in researching and developing practice, because it alludes to the methods and processes a researcher uses in order to attain higher levels of awareness and change strategies in relation to her foci of interest. As with many other research terms as it has become more mainstream reflexivity has been interpreted broadly especially within qualitative approaches to research. Nevertheless, it is important to try to grasp the essential meanings of the term if it is to be of practical use in discussions about reflective practice and research (Freshwater and Rolfe, 2001).

The role of the researcher in the research process has always been a contested issue. In quantitative (empirico-analytical) approaches, the researcher is directed by rigorously controlled methods to create and maintain objectivity within the project, so that the researcher's prejudices, emotions and intentions do not affect the data gathering and analysis phases, thereby ensuring the validity of the results. In contrast, qualitative research approaches tend to value the subjectivity of the researcher as a person who is involved inextricably in the research process yet is still able to remain self aware, thus ensuring that personal prejudices, emotions and intentions are not imposed on participants' accounts of their own experiences. Thus, despite many advances in thinking about and understanding research methods in recent years, there remains an objective-subjective divide between the two research traditions in relation to the role of the researcher. Discussions about researcher reflexivity attempt to shift the discussion towards a consideration of different epistemological perspectives, not only regarding the role of the researcher, but also about the types of knowledge that it is possible to generate and validate within human inquiry (Freshwater, Taylor and Sherwood, 2008).

Forms of reflexivity

Reflexivity is concerned essentially with the role of the researcher within the research process. No matter what the epistemological underpinnings, it is important to trace the different inflections that have been placed on the term in the practice and research literature. For example, over a decade ago Koch and Harrington (1998) identified four forms of reflexivity in relation to ethnography, suggesting that reflexivity could be understood:

- as being aimed at *sustaining objectivity* in the empirico-analytical tradition;
- as a means of *raising questions* about how knowledge is generated and validated through epistemology;
- from a *critical standpoint*, in which researchers locate themselves within political and social positions; and
- from a *feminist standpoint*, in which researchers embody and perform the politics of the researcher-participant relationship.

Reflexivity as a means of *raising questions* about how knowledge is generated and validated through epistemology also concerns itself with questions of context. This type of reflexivity examines how a research question is defined in order to explore an area of interest and the consequences of that definition on knowledge generation and validation processes and outcomes (Freshwater, Taylor and Sherwood, 2008). Epistemological reflexivity is based on the hermeneutics and writing of Hans Georg Gadamer (1975), who disputed Husserl's objective form of phenomenological reduction, claiming instead that humans are beings in the world through their lived experience; they cannot separate their being (ontology) from their knowing (epistemology) interests. The consequence for researchers of this type of reflexivity is a personal involvement in the research, in which they do not attempt to put their previous assumptions aside, but seek to leave themselves open to what might emerge in the study, so that they learn from the participants' accounts of their experiences.

As we have previously noted, from a *critical standpoint*, reflexivity involves researchers locating themselves within political and social positions, so that they remain mindful of the problematic nature of knowledge and power inherent in human relationships and organizations (Freshwater and Rolfe, 2001). Critical reflexivity draws particularly on the work and practice of the critical theory school of philosophy (see Chapter 3), which calls into question the socio-political structures in which we all find ourselves, and which reflects particularly on the effects of power, oppression and disempowerment in hegemonic situations.

From a *feminist standpoint*, reflexivity requires researchers to position themselves within an experiential location and to embody and perform the politics of the researcher–participant relationship in projects by and for women. Such feminist approaches reflect the 'reciprocal nature of the researcher-participant relationship' (Dowling, 2006), by examining potential and actual issues of differences in power, while maintaining engaged partnerships with participants.

Even though it is possible to categorize and apply various notions of reflexivity in this way, it is not easy to achieve involvement of participants in research projects without a degree of imposition. Many researchers acknowledge the difficulties experienced in recognizing their own taken for granted assumptions and values and the need to constantly reflect on how these might be surfaced. For example, some nurse researchers identify problems in attaining and maintaining reflexivity in clinical situations, where they may feel inclined to offer care in managing their emotional responses to the research participants' accounts (Pateman, 2000; Walsh-Bowers, 2002; Pellat, 2003; Allen, 2004; Whitehead, 2004).

Reflective moment

So far, the discussion might appear to be somewhat removed from clinical practice, and so this is a good moment at which to think about how your own practice has been influenced by research. Identify an area of your own practice that you would like to understand in more depth: how might you go about choosing the right research method? In choosing the appropriate method, think carefully about how this affects the role of the researcher and how the researcher might go about managing their own influences and interpretations and the subsequent impact of these on the findings.

In attempting to unpick the complexities of reflexivity and its relationship to reflection, sociologists such as Giddens (1984) have emphasized the interpretive nature of human knowledge and the monitored character of the ongoing flow of social life. As we have already noted, others see reflexivity in a more critical light, emphasizing opportunities for self-appraisal and critique within social contexts. These two positions on reflexivity reflect Taylor, Kermode and Roberts (2006) interpretive and critical categories of qualitative research, which will be discussed in more detail later.

Reflexivity and qualitative methodologies

Reflexivity is a fundamental consideration for qualitative researchers, both as a method and a process in a variety of methodologies, including ethnographic research and phenomenology (Koch and Harrington, 1998; Maich, Brown and Royle, 2000; Lenny, 2006), feminist research (Glass, 2000) and action research (Mantzoukas and Jasper, 2004). These methodologies vary in their emphasis on fundamental qualitative research assumptions about knowledge generation, such as giving voice, lived experience, subjectivity and intersubjectivity, context, and the intention to bring about change. They therefore use reflexivity differently to achieve their main intentions and to achieve methodological congruency.

Researchers using ethnographic and phenomenological methodologies regard reflexivity as a reflective process for exploring participants' lived experiences and documenting the researcher's role within the project, in order to prevent the imposition of researcher biases. In contrast, feminist researchers (Glass, 2000) view reflexivity as a thoughtful, shared process, bound inextricably to women's experiences, giving them voice and offering strategies to identify and transform oppressive situations. Action researchers (Mantzoukas and Jasper, 2004) acknowledge the power of reflection by using systematic critical questioning to identify and transform problematic social contexts that have previously been accepted as impervious to change.

Levels of participation vary, both across methods and across researchers. Reflexive researchers describe various levels of participation and involvement in the research process, from being an involved yet watchful participant observer, to being 'one of the others' as a co-researcher. The differing levels of involvement described here represent attempts to reduce the power differences between the researcher and the researched, and to increase the participants' sense of ownership of the project. These approaches also entail researchers documenting their reflections about their experiences as they participate on multiple levels of involvement within the research context. This reflexive transparency is intended to reduce the likelihood of imposing the researchers' preconceptions upon any aspect of the research and to explore the richness of intersubjective understandings of the research interests, thereby generating knowledge that informs the practice of nursing and health care (Freshwater, Taylor and Sherwood, 2008).

Reflective moment

Power is a key issue in any relationship, and is of particular concern when working in the caring professions. Researchers also have opportunities to exercise power and influence, since they work closely with vulnerable patients and colleagues whose professional resilience is tested on a daily basis. What are some of the key issues and considerations facing the reflective researcher when thinking about the potential power imbalance in the research situation?

It is fair to say that the thinking about reflection, its relationship to reflexivity and its role in research has moved on significantly since the first edition of this book, and arguably reflexivity can no longer be dismissed as a self-indulgent activity of 'navel gazing'. Rather, it is now commonly associated with methods and processes that enable researchers to explore their roles and influences within projects through systematic, critical questioning and appraisal. Even so, the involved yet non-imposing position sought by researchers within projects is not easy to attain and maintain, and thus researchers need to reflect constantly on their own roles and influences in order to bring participants' accounts of their experiences to the forefront.

Further reading

The following texts provide further reading on the topics covered in this chapter: Dowling (2006); Lenny (2006); Taylor (2008).

So far in this chapter, we have described the nature and forms of reflexivity and its important role in research. As we have already noted, we believe that reflection is fundamental to research, because thinking is fundamental to human life and inquiry. As Taylor, Kermode and Roberts (2006) note, 'Humans have the potential to think and to think about thinking, because we are endowed with the gifts of memory and reflection'. In research, thinking can take a variety of forms, such as reflecting on experiences, problem solving, inducing, deducing, synthesizing, interpreting and conceptualizing, all of which are linked inextricably to planning, doing, evaluating and disseminating research. Humans reflect as they review and contrast ideas and construct systematic approaches to human inquiry. With this fundamental principle in mind, we now describe, in brief, particular ways in which reflection and reflexivity can be used in research.

Paradigms and paradigm shifts

We saw in Chapter 2 that a paradigm can be described as an organizing framework for building knowledge and theory, including a view on what counts as knowledge, how it is generated and how it is to be disseminated. The dominant paradigm of a profession such as nursing therefore dictates and controls not only the content of professional knowledge, but also the processes by which that knowledge is produced (Malinski, 2002).

Researchers often categorize or group the various methodologies and epistemological approaches into quantitative and qualitative paradigms. In addition to, or perhaps beyond, these modernist classifications lies postmodernism that resists being reduced to a paradigm, even though it is seen by some writers as having been influential in shifting or upsetting traditional research categories. Thus, 'Postmodern thinking allows researchers to create highly imaginative research strategies to replace the relatively rigid rules and methods, that have been reflected in modernist (quantitative and some qualitative) research projects' (Freshwater, Taylor and Sherwood, 2008). Affirmative postmodern influences encourage researchers to move from their reliance on the 'scientific method' to be guided by their feelings, personal experience, empathy, emotion, intuition, subjective judgment, imagination, creativity and play. The inclusion of these subjective elements provokes a major departure from the rules of the 'scientific method' reflected in quantitative research, and constitutes an extension of qualitative researchers' ideas about the role of relative and personal knowledge in their projects.

Even though there has been a paradigm shift towards qualitative research and mixed methods research in nursing and other health professions, research driven from within the quantitative paradigm tends to dominate, not least because it attracts major funding from governments and health research sponsors. It is also seen to be more effective in supplying direct, objective facts about the causes, effects and treatment of human illnesses (Courtney, 2005). In essence, three major categories of research are used to generate and verify knowledge in health care; these are empirico-analytical, interpretive and critical approaches (Taylor, Kermode and Roberts, 2006).

Empirico-analytical research

Empirico-analytical research is concerned with observation, measurement and analysis through the application of the scientific method. The scientific method can be regarded as a set of rules and procedures that will guarantee valid and reliable research findings when applied in a rigorous manner. As we saw in Chapter 2, reliability can be defined simply as the production of consistently accurate findings over time and between researchers, and validity is achieved when the research tools can be demonstrated to measure or test what they set out to measure. In order to achieve validity and reliability, the scientific method demands that research be as free as possible from the distorting influences of the researcher, including the researcher's ideas, intentions and emotions (subjectivity). In other words, the researcher needs to show that due consideration has been given to achieving objectivity through the rigorous application of method. This process is traditionally regarded as the best way to build knowledge through inductive, deductive, theory-building, and theory-testing approaches, and is common to all disciplines that attempt or claim to produce scientific knowledge.

In addition, the scientific method requires that research questions be phrased and structured in ways that allow for empirical observation, numerical measurement and statistical analysis. For this reason, scientific researchers seek to reduce and simplify their objects of study to a set of variables that are amenable to quantitative manipulation and analysis (reductionism), often based on the underlying assumption that there are cause and effect links between certain objects and subjects. It is assumed that these cause and effect relationships have a far greater chance of being discovered if the variables in a study are carefully and objectively controlled and manipulated. Scientific researchers therefore take a great deal of care to design and implement their projects in a rigorous manner in order to ensure that they are observing and analyzing the effects of what they intend to study, so that they can demonstrate to the wider scientific community that the results are statistically significant. This means that they try to establish the degree of certainty they can place in cause and effect relationships through mathematical explanations.

Many of the health professions have sought to be identified as sciences by attaching importance to the use the empirico-analytical method for their research inquiry. For example, the discipline of nursing adopted this approach in the belief that it was the best way of developing nursing knowledge and of promoting the acceptance of nursing as a valid discipline. The quantitative scientific paradigm remains dominant in nursing and healthcare research, despite pressure from advocates of qualitative and postmodern approaches.

Interpretive and critical research

Given that qualitative research covers a vast conceptual area, it is convenient to divide the paradigm into interpretive and critical categories (Taylor, Kermode and Roberts, 2006). The main distinction between qualitative interpretive and qualitative critical research, is that interpretive researchers are concerned mainly with creating meaning, while critical researchers work collaboratively and systematically with co-researchers (participants) to identify issues, find solutions and use action strategies, to bring about emancipatory sociopolitical change. Qualitative research values humans and their experiences in the research process, and is concerned with questions that involve human consciousness and subjectivity. Qualitative research explores the changing (relative) nature of knowledge, which is centred on the people, place, time and conditions in which it finds itself (unique and context-dependent). Qualitative research starts from the specific instance and moves to the general pattern of combined instances (inductive), growing from the ground up to make wider statements about the nature of the thing being explored.

Rather than starting with a hypothesis, qualitative research usually begins with a general statement about the area of interest, such as: 'This research will explore the nature and effects of multidisciplinary team relationships in intensive care units'. The measures for ensuring validity in qualitative research involve asking the participants to confirm that the interpretations represent faithfully and clearly what the experience was/is like for them. Reliability or repeatability is often not an issue, as qualitative research is based on the assumption that knowledge reflects the unique features of the people, place, time and other circumstances (context) of the setting at the moment it was gathered. People are valued as sources of information and their expressions of their personal awareness (subjectivity) are seen as being integral to the meaning that arises from the research project. Unlike many quantitative approaches, qualitative research makes no claims to generate knowledge that can be confirmed through statistical means as certain (absolute).

Reflective practice fits well with qualitative research paradigms, since they share key assumptions about the value of the experiencing person within the research project, and each therefore regards lived experience, context and subjectivity as central concepts. This raises a problem for reflective research in terms of its status in generating evidence for health care, since the evidence-based practice movement places greatest value on evidence from quantitative research methods. In response to the demotion of qualitative research in general and reflective research in particular, a number of authors have critiqued evidence-based practice from various perspectives (Rolfe, 2001, 2003, 2005a, 2005b; Freshwater, 2004; Freshwater and Avis, 2004; Freshwater and Stickley, 2004; Jasper, 2005; Rolfe and Freshwater, 2005). Other critiques of the tendency of nursing to apply uncritically the ramifications of evidence-based practice focus on the implications it has for the establishment of new nursing roles (Jasper, 2005), the need to be clear conceptually about the sources, importance and effectiveness of levels of evidence (Rolfe, 2005a), and the dismissive responses by advocates of evidence-based practice towards thoughtful critiques of the movement (Rolfe, 2005b; Rolfe and Freshwater, 2005). Even so, paradigms have the power to resist change. As Freshwater, Taylor and Sherwood (2008) point out, 'evidence-based practice and the reflective practice paradigms are "grand narratives" that propose certain effective qualities in relation to nursing and health practice, but they do not have to be in opposition'.

Research approaches using reflection

Numerous possibilities exist for incorporating reflection in research, including

- storytelling,
- narrative,
- oral history,
- autobiographical methods,
- auto-ethnographical methods,
- action research,
- feminist research, and
- discourse analysis and discursive methods.

Storytelling and *narrative* are fundamental to reflective practice and research, because they involve a process of reflecting in order to recount and make sense of experiences (Holloway and Freshwater, 2007). The terms 'story', 'storying', 'storytelling' and 'narrative' have been used interchangeably. In an attempt to clarify the situation, Polkinghorne (1988) differentiated between a story as a single account intended to review life events in a true or imagined form, and a narrative as a scheme of multiple stories 'that organizes events and human actions into a whole'. Through research methods such as conversational interviews and reflective writing, stories can be gathered easily and effectively as people relate accounts of their lived experience. Making sense of the stories can be achieved through a variety of methods to best suit the research questions, aims and objectives. Oral history describes the past in a person's own words, which act as raw historical data, and which can stand alone as a single account, or be validated with and by other sources such as historical documents and photographs. Even though oral history has been viewed by some historians as marginal, suspect and trivial (Plummer, 1983), it is still promoted as a means of 'writing the individual back into collective memory' (Crane 1997).

The connections between oral history as a research approach and reflection as a process become apparent immediately, because the person giving the account of her life draws actively and systematically on cognitive processes to enable full descriptions of selected life aspects. *Autobiography* and *autoethnography* incorporate reflection and oral history, so can be used by people to retrace the events of their lives and the sense they have made of them through reflection.

Reflective moment

Think about your experience of listening to, telling and reading stories in day to day life. What makes a good story? What is the difference between a story that you read and one that is told? How does this relate to your experience of taking oral histories as a clinical procedure? Now think about the research that you have read in the past. What makes a good research story? How would you define or describe research that you find interesting and engaging to read?

Reflective processes and *action research* combine well to create effective collaborative qualitative research approaches for identifying and transforming clinical issues, because reflection is a key component of the action research method of planning, assessing, observing and reflecting. The discipline of nursing in particular recognizes the potential of reflective processes to improve practice through action research (Taylor, 2000; Thorpe and Barsky, 2001; Johns, 2003; Stickley and Freshwater, 2002), clinical supervision (Todd and Freshwater, 1999; Heath and Freshwater, 2000; Gilbert, 2001), education (Freshwater, 1999; Johns, 2000; Platzer, Blake and Ashford, 2000), and research (Freshwater and Rolfe, 2001; Taylor, 2001). Nursing is a complex practice involving knowledge, skills and human connection, so there are many opportunities for using reflection and action research as a collaborative research approach.

Action research involves four phases of collectively planning, acting, observing and reflecting. Each phase leads to another cycle of action, in which the plan is revised, and further acting, observing and reflecting is undertaken systematically, to work towards solutions to problems. The planning and acting phases may include any appropriate methods of gathering and analyzing data, such as participant observation, reflective journaling, surveys, focus groups and interviews. Cycles of action research lead to further foci and co-researchers can maintain an action research approach to their work for as long as they choose in order to find solutions to their practice problems. Feminism is a social movement concerned with women's issues and lives.

Feminist researchers agree that 'women are the major focus of feminist research from the beginning to the end of *whole* research projects'; therefore feminist methodology 'concerns research *by* and *for* women ... putting feminist theory into practice ... by applying feminist principles directly from feminist premises' (Glass, 2000). Feminist researchers generally choose the critical social theory paradigm as a means of personal empowerment of research participants, and this approach can be seen, for example, in the research projects of Lumby (1997), Boughton (2002), Tuttle and Seibold (2002) and Jackson et al. (2005).

As previously mentioned, the postmodern era continues to provide an eclectic extension to qualitative interpretive and critical research. Postmodernism resists being regarded as a third research paradigm, because postmodern thinking questions many of the taken-for-granted assumptions about knowledge generation and validation in research, and rejects taking on the authority of a 'grand narrative' ('big story' paradigm). Even so, it is possible to discuss postmodern influences on research methods and processes. Postmodernism seeks to upturn cherished notions of the importance of author, text, subject, history, time, theory, truth, representation and politics. It also requires researchers to redefine their basic assumptions, intentions and roles and to make adjustments to their present ways of viewing and doing research and practice.

This chapter can only provide the briefest of snapshots of approaches to research that can and do incorporate reflection as a fundamental concept within their methods and processes. However, it could be argued that all qualitative research is implicitly or explicitly reflective in nature, because its basic assumptions are that knowledge is generated and validated through people's lived experience as they give personal accounts of their subjective, contextualized experiences.

Reflective moment

Now turn back to the aims which you identified at the start of the chapter. To what extent have they been met? Write a paragraph outlining the factual and practical knowledge you have acquired through reading this chapter and doing the exercises. Write a second paragraph identifying any aims which you feel were only partially met or not met at all. As in the previous chapter, divide your page into three columns. Head the first column 'What I need to learn', and make a list of any outstanding issues which you would like to learn more about. For example, you might wish to find out more about practitioner research. Head the second column 'How I will learn it', and write down the ways in which your learning needs could be addressed; for example, through further reading, through attending study days, or through talking to other people. Head the third column 'How I will know that I have learnt it', and try to identify how you will know when you have met your needs.

10

Education and the reflective practitioner

Gary Rolfe

Introduction

As the health and social care professions moved one-by-one into the higher education sector during the second half of the twentieth century, the question of what professionals needed to know in order to practice began to take centre-stage. The educationalist Hazel Bines (1992) described the relocation of professional education from the site of practice to colleges and universities as the move from a pre-technocratic to a technocratic model of education characterized by 'the development and transmission of a systematic knowledge base... [and] the interpretation and application of the knowledge base to practice'. The term 'technocratic' thus refers to an educational model in which practice is driven by scientifically-derived theory, and where students are first taught this theory and only later are expected to apply it to practice. Prior to this time, most of the health and social care disciplines relied on an apprenticeship model of training, where the majority of the learning took place in an informal and unstructured way from practitioners at the site of practice, and much of the knowledge passed on in this way was tacit and heuristic.

However, the transition to a technocratic model brought with it a pressing need to develop a body of knowledge for the professions that was readily transmissible, generalizable and at the appropriate academic level. Since the pre-technocratic model of education dealt mostly in tacit knowledge that was difficult to put into words, the initial response of educationalists was to look elsewhere for the new systematic knowledge base for the health and social care professions. Depending on the requirements of each profession, this tended to be a mixture of the natural and social sciences, with much of the first wave of technocratic education being taught by academics from outside the professional discipline for which the students were being educated. This transition from pre-technocratic to technocratic education can be seen very clearly, for example, in the early *Project 2000* courses for nursing students in the 1990s, where new curricula were front-loaded with social and biological sciences, and where many of the nursing lecturers had no experience of teaching undergraduate students and did not themselves have university degrees. This situation is currently being repeated as other disciplines make the transition, and the knowledge-bases of the emerging professions are thus generally comprised of knowledge from other disciplines and professions, which is applied in a technocratic way to a discipline from which it was not itself derived.

As each profession begins to establish itself as an academic discipline in its own right, with all the trappings that this entails (journals, academic qualifications, and so on), it generally begins to take ownership of its knowledge-base. The 'pure' disciplines which formerly made up most of the taught input to students take on a more applied slant and begin to be taught by members of their own profession, and after a while a distinct professional knowledge-base begins to emerge. Finally, as professional disciplines become fully established in the higher education sector and the pressure to become academically and intellectually accepted becomes less urgent, attention is able to turn once again to practice and to the growing realization that a technocratic approach to education might be neither the most appropriate nor the most effective way of educating prospective and existing professional practitioners. We therefore find ourselves returning to the original aims of reflection expressed by John Dewey, David Kolb and others as *a way of learning* through experimenting with our environment. As Dewey (1938) very simply put it, 'we learn by doing and realizing what came from what we did'. The reflective practitioner is therefore continuously learning about practice through transforming the practice area into a site of *active learning* in which knowledge generation, knowledge acquisition and knowledge application are regarded as parts of a single process that we have referred to in this book as praxis.

While there have been many books written by and for educationalists which attempt to describe and discuss reflective education from the teacher's point of view, little has been written that addresses the needs and concerns of the reflective student. In this concluding chapter we shall therefore explore in more detail some of the implications of reflective learning for the health and social care practitioner and suggest ways in which you might maximize your learning from practice. While the majority of reflective learning takes place in and around the site of practice itself and goes largely unrecognized and unrewarded from an academic perspective, we shall also discuss some of the features you should look for in a formal academic course for reflective practitioners. The aims of this chapter are therefore:

1. to think about the ways in which you learn best;
2. to begin to map out your own learning needs and write learning plans to address them;
3. to consider critically a number of models of open learning; and
4. to help you to continue the process of lifelong learning.

Reflective moment

Think carefully about our aims for Chapter 10. Now think about your own practice and how these aims might contribute towards developing it.

Based on our aims above, identify and write down some aims of your own, both in terms of what you hope to know and what you hope to do after reading Chapter 10. We will return to these at the end of the chapter.

Learning from experience

In many ways, the turn to reflection as a way of constructing and articulating professional knowledge traces a full circle back to the pre-technocratic apprenticeship model of education, where the most important learning *about* practice occurs *in* practice and *from* practice. However, reflective education is firmly post-technocratic, insofar as it is a *response* to a technocratic model of education that has been found lacking when it comes to the needs of practice and practitioners. As Donald Schön put it, 'what aspiring practitioners most need to learn, professional schools seem least able to teach' (Schön 1987). As Schön pointed out, the classroom and the skills laboratory can only take us so far with professional education, since neither fully prepares the student to deal with the messy and unpredictable world of practice. Sooner or later, both the educator and the student must acknowledge 'neither that existing professional knowledge fits every case nor that every problem has a right answer' (Schön 1987). The most important difference between the pre-technocratic and the technocratic approaches on the one hand, and the reflective post-technocratic approach on the other, lies in the acknowledgement by the latter of the practitioner's own knowledge-base. Whereas the traditional apprenticeship model regards practice knowledge as mostly hidden and largely inexpressible, and whereas the technocratic model regards practice knowledge as largely irrelevant, the reflective model places the construction of knowledge from experience at its heart.

This post-technocratic model, which assumes that the most appropriate knowledge for practice is located not in books nor even in universities, but in practice itself, presents a number of challenges for educationalists and curriculum writers. As Boud, Keogh and Walker, (1985) pointed out:

> Only learners themselves can learn and only they can reflect on their own experiences. Teachers can intervene in various ways to assist, but they only have access to individuals' thoughts and feelings through what individuals choose to reveal about themselves. At this basic level the learner is in total control. (1985, p. 11)

Clearly, then, the educationalist has a very different role to play in the post-technocratic model than in traditional passive learning. Indeed, as Boud, Keogh and Walker (1985) implied above, the role of the *teacher* is largely redundant.

This does not mean that the university or college lecturer has no place in the education of the reflective practitioner, but simply that her role is not to teach in the traditional sense of delivering knowledge and theory. Rather, she is concerned with facilitating the practitioner to construct, gain access to, and critically explore her own experiential knowledge from her own practice. Just as the practitioner is an expert in the practice and process of health and social care, so the educationalist should be an expert in the practice and process of education. What the educationalist possesses that the healthcare practitioner does not, is experiential knowledge about the process of learning; to return to the distinction that we made in Chapter 2, it is not 'knowing-that' that is important in post-technocratic education, but 'knowing-how'. The post-technocratic educationalist knows *how* to enable the practitioner to learn from their own experience.

Post-technocratic reflective education is therefore concerned far more with process than with content. This distinction is particularly important in the education of more experienced or advanced practitioners, since it removes the necessity for the educator to possess more 'know-how' about health and social care practice than the practitioner herself. The role of the educator is not to teach the practitioner how to practice, but to help her to learn from her own reflections on her own practice. Of course, the practitioner might also need access to factual scientific knowledge, but it is not the job of the educator to tell her what she needs to know, but rather to help her to seek out, gain access to, and evaluate the relevant published material. Seen in this way, the health and social care practitioner and the practitioner of education form a partnership of equals, each with their own expertise in their own realm of practice.

Reflective moment

One of the great advantages of post-technocratic education is that it allows the student to plan her own learning based on her own particular needs and strengths. The psychologist Donald Kolb (1984) identified four distinct learning styles as follows:

- Divergent learners are imaginative and capable of viewing situations from a variety of perspectives. They are 'feelers' rather than 'doers', and are good at brainstorming new ideas.
- Convergent learners are good at abstract conceptualization and active experimentation. They prefer technical problems to interpersonal issues, and are adept at scientific or hypothetical-deductive reasoning.
- Assimilative learners also tend towards abstract conceptualization, but they are observers rather than doers. They are good at inductive reasoning and are able to create theoretical models and assimilate disparate observations into an integrated explanation.
- Accommodative learners have the opposite strengths to assimilative learners, and are interested in concrete experience and active experimentation. Their greatest strength lies in doing things, in carrying out plans and tasks, and in getting involved in new experiences.

Think about how you learn best and try to identify which learning style you feel most comfortable with. Now think about how your learning style might translate into particular ways of learning, for example, working in a group, attending lectures or working from books.

Further reading

To find out more about Kolb's model of learning, see Kolb (1984). A simplified version of his Learning Style Inventory can be found in Kolb, Osland and Rubin (1995). For an easy-to-read overview of Kolb's work on reflective learning and learning styles, see Chapter 4 of MacKeracher (2004).

In this book, we have offered a number of approaches to active experiential learning, including writing-to-learn (Chapter 5), individual and group supervision (Chapters 6 and 7) and reflection-in-action (Chapter 8). We now wish to distil these approaches into a process model of learning, first for the post-technocratic reflective and reflexive practitioner in order to help her to become a lifelong learner, and second for the post-technocratic educationalist in order to help her to think more creatively about curriculum design.

The educational journey

Education has often been described as a journey, and it might be instructive to compare the metaphorical educational journey with a real journey from one place to another. For example, we might think about what happens when we stop someone in the street and ask her for help in getting to our destination. There are essentially three ways that a passer-by might offer help if I am lost: first, she might personally take me to where I want to go; second, she might give me directions (for example, take the first road on the left, turn right at the traffic lights, etc.); and third, she might draw a map for me.

Similarly, there are three main ways to get from A to B in education. First, the educator can personally take the student. This is usually known as the apprenticeship model, or what Bines (1992) earlier referred to as pre-technocratic education, and involves the student working alongside a more experienced educator/practitioner or practice teacher. The apprenticeship model is the basis of most traditional courses in professional education, but is now usually thought of as being too *ad hoc* and unacademic for most professions. It can be successful, but depends largely on the educational skills and qualities of the practitioner. Furthermore, it lacks a formal structure and relies primarily on the gradual and largely unconscious absorption of skills by the student. Rather like being driven along an unknown route, the student tends not to pay too much attention to the route, and probably could not retrace alone.

Second, the educator could give directions to the student in the form of a syllabus backed up with lectures and set reading, with an examination or other form of assessment to check whether the route has been followed. This is Bines' model of technocratic education, and is the foundation of most modern courses in professional education such as *Project 2000* for pre-registration nurses that we mentioned earlier, and many taught post-qualifying courses. The implicit or (sometimes) explicit aim of such courses is not to learn what the student finds interesting or relevant, but what is set out in the syllabus. This sends a clear message to the student that the educator knows best what they need to learn, and usually how best they might learn it. The aim when writing assignments and revising for examinations is therefore to attempt to guess the 'right' answers, that is, the answers dictated by the syllabus. While this model might be appropriate for neophyte practitioners, it is clearly arrogant of the educator to assume that she knows best what the experienced or advanced practitioner needs to learn, and indeed, how it might best be learnt.

Third, the educator can give the student a map. This is a fairly recent approach to learning, what Bines referred to as 'post-technocratic' education and what others have referred to as 'open learning', and it gives the student a degree of control over how to get from A to B. She still has to get there (usually there are still learning outcomes to be achieved), but there is some degree of choice about which route to take, and sometimes about the precise location of point B. As we shall see, this post-technocratic model is most appropriate for reflective and reflexive practitioners.

Reflective moment

Think about a previous course you have been on. Try to identify which of the three educational models described above was mainly employed. With a colleague, discuss the things you liked and disliked about that approach. How did it suit your style of learning?

A map of professional practice

At the start of his book *Educating the Reflective Practitioner,* Donald Schön observed that:

In the varied topography of professional practice, there is a high, hard ground overlooking a swamp. On the high ground, manageable problems lend themselves to solution through the application of research-based theory and technique. In the swampy lowland, messy, confusing problems defy technical solution. The irony of this situation is that the problems of the high ground tend to be relatively unimportant to individuals or society at large, however great their technical interest may be, while in the swamp lie the problems of greatest human concern. The practitioner must choose. Shall he remain on the high ground where he can solve relatively unimportant problems according to prevailing standards of rigor, or shall he descend to the swamp of important problems and nonrigorous inquiry? (Schön, 1987, p. 3)

Schön suggests that these 'messy confusing problems [that] defy technical solution', can only be explored through reflective and reflexive practice. The problem is that few educationalists are qualified or experienced to take the more advanced practitioner through the swamp from A to B themselves, and providing a list of directions is hardly appropriate at this level, even supposing that the educator had enough experiential knowledge to compile one. It clearly makes far more sense to give the student a map of the terrain so that they can plot their own route.

We have seen that a list of educational directions might take the form of a traditional curriculum, but what, we might ask ourselves, would an educational map look like? It is perhaps easier to say what it would *not* look like. An educational map would not present the student with a sequential list of outcomes and objectives, nor with set reading or compulsory lectures. It would not prescribe a single route for getting from A to B and might not even specify where B is located. More importantly, a map can show uncharted territory; places that the educationalist has not visited; indeed, places where no one has visited. In this sense, the student is able to get more information out of an educational map than was originally put into it, inasmuch as it allows the student to go to places that were never intended (or even envisaged) by the map maker.

Mapping out your learning needs

The purpose of an educational map is to help you to plan your own learning path from A to B. However, in order to extract information from a map, you need to know how to read it, and this is where an educationalist can be of help. In order to read a map, you need first to know its scale. At one extreme, educational maps can show the entire landscape of a professional career, while at the other, they can provide great detail about very specific learning needs. In planning your reflective education, you need both. On the one hand you need an overview of your career in order to plan where you want to be in (say) 10 years time, but on the other hand you need to zoom in on your specific learning for the next six months, or even the next week.

If you are to use the map in order to move forwards, there are four factors that you will need to consider. First, you will need to determine just where on the map you currently are. What is your present location in terms of qualifications, experience or job title? What is the current state of your knowledge and experience of a particular issue? Second, you will need to decide where you wish to go. Your destination might be Schön's high, hard ground of technical specialism, of management, or of education, or it might be out in the swampy lowlands building your experiential knowledge and becoming a more reflective or reflexive practitioner. On a micro level, you need to identify your immediate learning needs in order to take the next step towards your long-term macro level goals. Third, you will need to decide how you are going to get there. Do you wish to travel along the quickest or the most scenic route? Perhaps you are taking a particular course purely out of interest, even though it will not be of any practical use in furthering your career. What is your favoured mode of transport; that is, when, where and how do you learn best? Which of Kolb's four learning styles suits your needs? Do you need structured learning experiences such as lectures or self-directed ones such as reading or reflecting on practice? Fourth, you will need some way of identifying when you have arrived. If your chosen destination is a particular job or qualification, there will be some familiar landmarks to signal your arrival. If, on the other hand, you have chosen to remain in the swamp and develop your experiential knowledge, then it might not be quite so obvious that you have arrived. Just as importantly, how will you be able to demonstrate to others that you have reached your destination?

Figure 10.1 A framework for a simple learning plan

Learning plan

- What do I already know?
- What do I want to learn?
- How do I want to learn it?
- How will I know, and be able to demonstrate, that I have learnt

If we put these four issues together – identifying the current state of your knowledge and theory; deciding what it is that you want and need from education; planning how these wants and needs are going to be met; and identifying how you will know that your wants and needs have been met – we have the framework for a simple learning plan (Figure 10.1).

Learning plans are the basis for lifelong learning, and can help you to achieve both your short- and long-term goals. Learning plans might be made in conjunction with an educationalist as part of a formal course, or else they might be made solely by the practitioner. You have probably noticed that each chapter of this book ends by asking you to assess what you have learnt from reading it (What do I already know?), to identify what other knowledge you still need (What do I want to learn?), how you might go about obtaining it (How do I want to learn it?), and how you will know that you have achieved it (How will I know, and be able to demonstrate, that I have learnt it?). If you have carried out these exercises, you have therefore written a series of learning plans to give structure and direction to your individual lifelong learning about reflective practice.

Reflective moment

Draw a map of your current practice in whatever style you choose. It might take the form of a 'road map' of your career or a 'mind map' for a specific learning need. It might be pictorial or textual, abstract or concrete, literal or figurative. Try to be imaginative and include as much detail as you can. Now identify where you are on your map, and think about your next destination. What is your most immediate educational need in moving towards your goal?

Using the above format, try to write a learning plan to meet part of that need. For example, you might identify the need to learn more about evidence-based practice, and choose to write a learning plan to help you to conduct a systematic literature review.

An open learning course for reflective and reflexive practitioners

As well as using learning plans to identify and structure your individual learning needs, they can also be agreed and negotiated with an educationalist as part of a formal and accredited open learning course. The term 'open learning' is often misused, partly because it is sometimes confused with the term 'distance learning'. The former is a philosophy of education, whereas the latter is a way of delivering what can be (and often is) a very traditional 'closed' course. The purpose of open learning courses is not to tell you what or how you should be learning, but to give you access to some experienced educational map-makers who can offer help and advice on plotting your own route through a series of learning plans. Open learning can be undertaken at any level from primary school to post-doctoral study, but our concern here is with exploring some of the key features of an undergraduate or post-graduate open learning course for reflective and reflexive practitioners. The structure of a learning plan for an open-learning course poses the same four questions as for informal reflective learning. These questions have been formulated be asked by a practitioner in attempting to choose an open learning course, but are also relevant for an educationalist to help her to think about designing one.

What do I already know?

To continue our map analogy, the first question to be addressed in the learning plan is the equivalent of establishing point A (where am I now?) on the map. Unlike in the examples of being taken or of being given directions to your destination, it is essential when reading a map to know where you are at the moment, that is, the current state of your knowledge and practice. Furthermore, this is likely to be something that is different for each student, and all that most post-qualifying health and social care students have in common is that they each bring a unique and individual body of theoretical and practical knowledge with them to a course. Traditional courses assume or require that all the students are at more or less the same point on starting, whereas open learning courses work with the student in order to help her to identify her own starting point.

What do I want to learn?

The second question in the learning plan is concerned with deciding on the location of point B. Unlike on most traditional courses, where your learning destination is established in advance by the syllabus and the course assignments, open learning usually requires you to decide where it is on the map that you wish to go. By writing a learning plan, the student is therefore to some extent writing her own course syllabus.

One of the difficulties with taking such an open approach to course design is that the student is often spoilt for choice: with so many learning needs, so many potential destinations, it is difficult to make decisions about which is the most pressing. In attempting to resolve this problem, we should always bear in mind the first tenet of experiential learning; that the most important and meaningful learning arises from the challenges raised by practice. It is only when undertaking a new project that the practitioner runs up against the limitations of her own knowledge and understanding, just as it is only when we move out of our own familiar locality that we have to stop and consult our map. Ideally, then, open learning courses for reflective practitioners should be project-based, since it is only through planning and implementing new practice-based projects that the practitioner can begin to identify the learning needed in order to support and carry out that project. Since most practitioners are very busy people, courses should be based largely around *real* projects that they have recently completed, are currently involved in, or are about to commence.

How do I want to learn it?

The third question asks you to decide on your mode of transport. To some extent, different kinds of knowledge are best acquired by particular methods of learning. Some knowledge (for example, scientific theoretical knowledge) is most easily and appropriately learnt in a classroom from an expert in that particular kind of knowledge or else from reading a book. Other kinds of knowledge (for example, experiential practical knowledge) can only be learnt from other practitioners or from yourself through discussion and reflection-on-action, and it should be borne in mind that learning *about* practice often means learning *from* practice, and for the reflective practitioner, that usually means learning from her own practice.

However, although different kinds of knowledge lend themselves to different forms of learning, most students also have their favoured style. Some learn best in a classroom, some from private study, some from reflective writing and some from group discussions and seminars. In open learning courses, then, the student should have a large degree of freedom in deciding exactly how she will get from A to B; that is, on *how* she wishes to learn as well as *what* she wishes to learn.

How will I know, and be able to demonstrate, that I have learnt it?

Finally, the fourth question is concerned with verifying that you actually are at point B where you think you are. The simple answer to this question is that you write an assignment that is marked by a tutor. In traditional courses, where the destination is set in advance by the syllabus, the assessment often drives the course, and the first question that most new students ask is 'what do I need to do in order to pass this course?' In open learning courses, the assessment depends on the location of point B and the mode of transport employed in order to get there, and will often be decided by the student herself.

The more complex answer to the question concerns the nature of the assignment, particularly when the course is centred on a practice-based project. We have already asserted that open learning involves collaboration between an experienced practitioner and an experienced educationalist, each with their own specific experiential and theoretical knowledge. However, if the educationalist is an expert in education rather than in health and social care practice, then there are very real concerns surrounding the expert's ability to assess the practice-based work of the practitioner. Indeed, it might be argued that the person best placed to assess practice-based projects is the practitioner herself.

Figure 10.2 Some questions to ask about open learning courses for reflective practitioners

- Is the course structured through learning plans negotiated between the practitioner and an educationalist?
- Is it organised around real practice-based projects in the practitioner's own workplace?
- Does it offer access to a wide range of taught and self-directed learning opportunities of relevance to each individual practitioner?
- Does it facilitate and encourage the practitioner to explore her experiential knowledge-base through reflection-on-action?
- Does it facilitate the practitioner to critically evaluate her own project work?
- Does it facilitate the sharing of knowledge and experience between practitioners, both within and outside of the practitioner's own specialism, through seminars, discussions and group work?
- Is it structured to fit the busy schedule of the practitioner rather than that of the educationalist?
- Does it promote a relationship between practitioner and education-alist as a partnership of equals, each with skills, knowledge and expertise in their own discipline?

This notion of critical self-appraisal fits perfectly with the philosophy of open learning, which should be concerned not only with self-education, but also with self-evaluation. Indeed, it could be argued that self-evaluation is the highest-level cognitive skill and the most difficult to master. The role of the educationalist should therefore be to provide the knowledge and theory to enable the reflective practitioner to critically evaluate her own practice-based projects, and to support and facilitate her through the process. Of course, there is still a requirement on most academic courses for the assignment to be marked and accredited by an educationalist, but her role is now to assess the practitioner's evaluation of her own project rather than directly to evaluate the project herself. This approach separates assessment (which is the job of the educationalist) from evaluation (which is the job of the reflective practitioner), so that what is required from an assignment is not necessarily a successful project, but a skilled and critical evaluation, even of an unsuccessful project.

We can see, then, that open learning courses are likely to look very different from more traditional taught courses, and some of the questions you might wish to ask when choosing or designing such a course are suggested in Figure 10.2.

Reflective moment

Try to imagine what an open learning course of this type would be like, and how it might be structured. With a colleague, discuss some of the pros and cons of such a course.

It is unlikely that any course will meet all of the criteria suggested in Table 10.2, and perhaps not all will be appropriate to your own needs. However, it is important that you have your own shopping list when looking at prospective courses.

As a prospective student, think about what issues are important to you in an open learning course. Write down your own list of questions that you would wish to ask the tutor of a course that you might apply for.

As an educationalist, think about what issues are important to you in designing an open learning course. Write down a list of educational principles on which you would base such a course.

Further reading

If you would like to read more about open learning, you might like to start with the seminal work of Carl Rogers (1983) (who referred to it as student-centred learning) and Malcolm Knowles (1984) (who referred to it as andragogy), who are usually acknowledged as the modern-day founders of this approach. Gould and Taylor (1996) have written a useful guide to reflective learning for social workers, Rideout (2001) has produced something similar for nurses, and Brockbank and McGill's (2007) book is aimed more generally at teachers in higher education, also see Davies (2008).

Conclusion: becoming a lifelong learner

Since the development of our practice is a lifelong endeavour, then so too is our learning. For reflective and reflexive practitioners, the two activities cannot be separated: the very act of reflecting on and in practice generates knowledge, and so to practice is also to learn (and, indeed, to research).

In many ways, then, this entire book has been concerned with learning: through critical reflection, through reflective writing, through individual and group supervision, through reflection-in-action and through reflective research. However, in most of these activities the learning is *ad hoc* and often secondary to some other goal such as developing practice or doing research. In this chapter we have focused on learning as an end in itself, and discussed some of the ways that the reflective and reflexive practitioner can structure her learning experiences either informally or through a formal taught course.

The most important learning, however, is what we might call meta-learning, that is, learning about how you learn. This meta-learning is the basis of lifelong learning. If we help a practitioner to learn about (say) depressive illness and to work with people suffering from depressive illness, then we have equipped her to carry out a task for a limited time-span until her knowledge and skills become outdated. However, if we help a practitioner to learn how to learn, then we have equipped her for life by providing her with the tools to develop her own knowledge through reflection in- and on-action, through reflexive research and through open learning. Critical reflective practice, or what we have referred to as *praxis*, can therefore be seen as a paradigm of practice, an organizing framework for building knowledge and theory, including a philosophy about what counts as knowledge and the practical tools for generating and applying it to practice.

Let us return once more to our map analogy. If we take a traveller to where she wants to go, or if we give her directions, we will help her to reach her next destination but no further. If we give her a map, she will be able to navigate without further help until she comes to the edge of that map or until the map becomes out of date. If, on the other hand, we show her how to make her own maps, then she can continue with her travels for as long and as far as she wishes. We regard praxis as a process of exploring previously uncharted areas of practice and making maps of it as you go along. Our hope is that, having read this book, you have begun to sketch out your first maps and will continue to work on refining them throughout your life as a practitioner. Do remember, though, that in the words of the scientist and philosopher Alfred Korzybski (1995), 'The map is not the territory', and ultimately it is the territory of practice, out there in Donald Schön's 'swampy lowland', where health and social care practice makes a real difference to real people.

Reflective moment

Now turn back to the aims which you identified at the start of the chapter. To what extent have they been met? Write a paragraph outlining the scientific and experiential knowledge you have acquired through reading this chapter and doing the exercises. Write a second paragraph identifying any aims which you feel were only partially met or not met at all. Now divide your page into three columns. Head the first column 'What I need to learn', and make a list of any outstanding issues which you would like to learn more about. Head the second column 'How I will learn it', and write down the ways in which your learning needs could be addressed, for example, through further reading, through attending study days, or through talking to other people. Head the third column 'How I will know that I have learnt it', and try to identify how you will know when you have met your needs.

You have just written the last learning plan of this book, but not, we hope, the last of your career.

References

Adair, J. (2005) *How to Grow Leaders*, London, Kogan Page.

Alcauskas, M. and Charon, R (2008) 'Right Brain: Reading, Writing, and Reflecting: Making a Case for Narrative Medicine in Neurology', *Neurology*, 70.

ALG (Action Learning Group, West Midlands) (2006) Birmingham, Pers. Com.

Allen, D. (2004) 'Ethnomethodological Insights into Insider-Outsider Relationships in Nursing Ethnographies of Healthcare Settings', *Nursing Inquiry*, 11(1).

Allen, D.G., Bowers, B. and Diekelmann, N. (1989) 'Writing to Learn: A Reconceptualization of Thinking and Writing in the Nursing Curriculum', *Journal of Nursing Education*, 28(1).

Alleyne, J.O. and Jumaa, M.O. (2007) 'Building the Capacity for Evidence-Based Clinical Nursing Leadership', *Journal of Nursing Management*, 15.

Alterio, M (2004) 'Collaborative Journalling as a Professional Development Tool', *Journal of Further and Higher Education*, 28(3).

Arvidsson, B., Lofgren, H. and Fridland, B. (2001) 'Psychiatric Nurses' Conceptions of How a Group Supervision Programme in Nursing Care Influences their Professional Competence: A 4 year Follow-Up Study', *Journal of Nursing Management*, 9.

Atkins, S. and Murphy, K. (1994) 'Reflective Practice', *Nursing Standard*, 8(39).

Barker, P. (2007) *Basic Family Therapy*, 5th edn, Oxford, Blackwell.

Benner, P. (1984) *From Novice to Expert*, Reading, MA, Addison-Wesley.

Berstein, S. (ed.) (1965) *Explorations in Groupwork*, Boston, MA, Boston University Press.

Bertcher, H.J. (1994) *Group Participation Techniques for Leaders and Members*, 2nd edn, Thousand Oaks, Sage.

Bines, H. (1992) 'Issues in Course Design', in Bines and Watson (1992).

Bines, H. and Watson, D. (eds) (1992) *Developing Professional Education*, Buckingham, Open University Press.

Bion, W.R. (1989) *Experiences in Groups and Other Papers*, London, Tavistock/Routledge.

Bishop, V. (ed) (2006) *Clinical Supervision*, 2nd edn, Basingstoke, Palgrave.

Bockbank, A. and McGill, I. (2007) *Facilitating Reflective Learning in Higher Education*, 2nd edn, Maidenhead, Open University Press.

Bolton, G. (2005) *Reflective Writing*, 2nd edn, London, Paul Chapman.

Bolton, G (2006) 'Narrative Writing: Reflective Enquiry into Professional Practice', *Educational Action Research*, 14(2).

Bond, T. (1986) *Games for Social and Life Skills*, London, Hutchinson.

Bond, M. and Holland, S. (1998) *Skills of Clinical Supervision for Nurses*, Buckingham, Open University Press.

Borton, T. (1970) *Reach, Touch and Teach*, London, McGraw-Hill.

Boud. D., Cohen, R. and Walker, D. (2000) *Using Experience for Learning*. Buckingham, Open University Press.

Boud, D., Keogh, R. and Walker, D. (1985) *Reflection: Turning Experience into Learning*, London, Kogan Page.

Boughton, M. (2002) 'Premature Menopause: Multiple Disruptions between a Woman's Biological Body Experience and Her Lived Body', *Journal of Advanced Nursing*, 37(5).

Bowers, S. and Jinks, A. (2004) 'Issues Surrounding Professional Portfolio Development for Nurses', *British Journal of Nursing*, 13(3).

Boychuk Duchscher, J.E. (1999) 'Catching the Wave: Understanding the Concept of Critical Thinking', *Journal of Advanced Nursing*, 29 (3).

Boyd, E. and Fales, A. (1983) 'Reflective Learning: The Key to Learning from Experience', *Journal of Humanistic Psychology*, 23(2).

Brady, D., Corbie-Smith, G. and Branch, W. (2002) '"What's Important to You?": The Use of Narratives to Promote Self-Reflection and To Understand the Experiences of Medical Residents', *Annals of Internal Medicine, American College of Physicians*, 137(3).

Brandes, D. (1984) *Gamesters' Handbook Two*, London, Hutchinson.

Brandes, D. and Norris, J. (1998) *Gamesters' Handbook Three*, London, Hutchinson.

Brandes, D. and Phillips, H. (1979) *Gamesters' Handbook*, London, Hutchinson.

Brodie, L (2007) 'Reflective Writing by Distance Education Students in an Engineering Problem Based Learning Course', *Australasian Journal of Engineering Education*, 13(2).

Brookfield, S.D. (1987) *Developing Critical Thinkers: Challenging Adults to Explore Alternative Ways of Thinking and Acting*, San Francisco, Jossey Bass.

Brookfield, S.D. (1995) *Becoming a Critically Reflective Teacher*, San Francisco, Jossey-Bass.

Brown, A. (1984) *Consultation for Social Workers*, London, Heinemann Educational.

Brown, A. (1989) *Groupwork*, 2nd edn, Aldershot, Gower.

Bullock, A. Stallybrass, O. Trombley, S. and Eadie, B. (eds) (1988) *The Fontana Dictionary of Modern Thought*, London, HarperCollins.

Bulman, C. and Burns, S. (eds) (2000) *Reflective Practice in Nursing*, 2nd edn, Oxford, Blackwell Scientific.

Bulman, C. and Schutz, S. (eds) (2008) *Reflective Practice in Nursing*, 4th edn, Oxford, Blackwell.

Burnham, J.B. (1986) *Family Therapy*, London, Tavistock Publications.

Burr, V. (1995) *An Introduction to Social Constructionism*, London, Routledge.

Burton, A.J. (2000) Reflection: Nursing's Practice and Education Panacea? *Journal of Advanced Nursing*, 31(5).

Butterworth, T. and Faugier, J. (eds) (1992) *Clinical Supervision and Mentorship in Nursing*, London, Chapman Hall.

Butterworth, T. and Faugier, J. (eds) (1998) *Clinical Supervision and Mentorship in Nursing*, Cheltenham, Stanley Thornes.

Cardinal, D., Hayward, J. and Jones, G. (2004) *Epistemology: The Theory of Knowledge*, London, John Murray.

Carper, B.A. (1978) 'Fundamental Patterns of Knowing in Nursing', *Advances in Nursing Science*, 1(1): 13–23.

Carr, W. and Kemmis, S. (1986) *Becoming Critical*, London, Falmer Press.

Carroll, M., Curtis, L., Higgins, A., Nicholl, H., Redmond, R., and Timmins, F. (2002) 'Is There a Place for Reflective Practice in the Nursing Curriculum?', *Nurse Education in Practice*, 2(1).

Cartwright, D. and Zander, A. (eds) (1968) *Group Dynamics*, 3rd edn, New York, Harper & Row.

Casement, P. (1985) *On Learning from the Patient*, London, Tavistock.

Charon, R. (2001) 'Narrative Medicine: A Model for Empathy, Reflection, Profession, and Trust', *Journal of American Medical Association*, 286(15).

Chirema, K. (2007) 'The Use of Reflective Journals in the Promotion of Reflection and Learning in Post-Registration Nursing Students', *Nurse Education Today*, 27.

Cleary, M. and Freeman, A. (2005) 'The Cultural Realities of Clinical Supervision in an Acute Inpatient Mental Health Setting', *Issues in Mental Health Nursing*, 26.

Clouder, L. and Sellars, J. (2004) 'Reflective Practice and Clinical Supervision: An Interprofessional Perspective', *Journal of Advanced Nursing*, 46(3).

Cole, M.B. (2005) *Group Dynamics in Occupational Therapy*, 3rd edn, Thorofare, CA, SLACK Incorporated.

Cole, P. (2002) *The Theory of Knowledge*, London, Hodder & Stoughton.

Comte, A. (1988) *Introduction to Positive Philosophy*, Indianapolis, Hackett Publishing.

Courtney, M. (Ed) (2005) *Evidence for Nursing Practice*, Sydney, Elsevier Churchill Livingstone.

Cowan, J. (2006) *On Becoming an Innovative University Teacher: Reflection-in-action*, 2nd edn, Maidenhead, Open University Press.

Cox, C. (2002) *Enhancing the Practice Experience*, London, Praxis.

Cox, H., Hickson, P. and Taylor, B. (1991) 'Exploring Reflection: Knowing and Constructing Practice', in Gray and Pratt (1991).

Crane, S. (1997) 'Writing the Individual Back into Collective Memory', *American Historical Review*, 110.

Cunliffe, A.L. (2004) 'On Becoming a Critically Reflexive Practitioner', *Journal of Management Education*, 28, 4.

Curtise, K., White, P. and McKay, J (2008) 'Establishing a Method to Support Academic and Professional Competence throughout an Undergraduate Radiography Programme', *Radiography*, 14.

Dartington, A. (1994) 'Where Angels Fear to Tread: Idealism, Despondency and Inhibition of Thought in Hospital Nursing', in Obholzer and Roberts (1994).

Davies, L. (2008) *Informal Learning: A New Model for Making Sense of Experience*, Aldershot, Gower.

DeMarco, R., Rosanna, F., Roberts, S. and Chandler, G (2005) 'The Use of a Writing Group to Enhance Voice and Connection Among Staff Nurses', *Journal for Nurses in Staff Development*, 21(3).

Department of Health (1993) *A Vision for the Future: The Nursing, Midwifery and Health Visiting Contribution to Health and Health Care*, London, HMSO.

Dewey, J. (1938) *Experience and Education*, New York, Macmillan.

Douglas, T. (2000) *Basic Groupwork*, 2nd edn, London, Routledge.

Dowling, M. (2006) 'Approaches to Reflexivity in Qualitative Research', *Nurse Researcher*, 13(3).

Dreyfus, H.L. and Dreyfus, S.E. (1986) *Mind Over Machine*, Oxford, Basil Blackwell.

Driscoll, J. (2000) *Practising Clinical Supervision*, London, Balliere Tindall.

Ennis, R.H. (1985) 'A Logical Basis for Measuring Critical Thinking Skills', *Educational Leadership*, 43(2).

Enyedy, K C , Arcinye, F., Puri, N.N., Carter, J.W., Goodyear, R.K. and Getzelman, M.A. (2003) 'Hindering Phenomena in Group Supervision: Implications for Practice', *Professional Psychology: Research and Practice*, 34.

Eraut, M. (1994) *Developing Professional Knowledge and Competence*, London, Falmer Press.

Eraut, M. (2004) 'The Practice of Reflection', *Learning in Health and Social Care*, 3.

Espeland, K. and Shafa, L. (2001) 'Empowering versus Enabling in Academia', *Journal of Nursing Education*, 40(8).

Esterhuizen, P. and Freshwater, D. (2008) 'Clinical Supervision and Reflective Practice', in Freshwater, Taylor and Sherwood.

Evans, T. and Hardy, M. (2010) *Evidence and Knowledge for Practice*, Cambridge, Polity Press.

Evidence-Based Medicine Working Group (1992) 'Evidence-Based Medicine: A New Approach to Teaching the Practice of Medicine', *JAMA*, 268(17).

Facione, P.A. (1990) *The Delphi Report. Critical Thinking: A Statement of Expert Consensus for Purposes of Educational Assessment and Instruction. Executive Summary*, Millbrae California, The California Academic Press.

Facione, P.A., Facione, N.C. and Sanchez, C.A. (1994) 'Critical Thinking Disposition as a Measure of Competent Clinical Judgement: The Development of the California Critical Thinking Disposition Inventory', *Journal of Nursing Education*, 33.

Faugier, J. (1992) 'The Supervisory Relationship', in Butterworth and Faugier (1992).

Faugier, J. and Butterworth, T. (1994) *Clinical Supervision: A Position Paper*, Manchester, University of Manchester.

Fiedler, F.E. (1981) *Leader Attitudes and Group Effectiveness*, Westport, CT, Greenwood.

Fitzgerald, M. (1994) Theories of Reflection for Learning, in Palmer, Burns and Bulman (1994).

Fitzgerald, M. (2000) Clinical Supervision and Reflective Practice, in Bulman and Burns (2000).

Flanagan, J. (1954) 'The Critical Incident Technique', *Psychological Bulletin*, 51(4).

Forsyth, D.R. (2010) *Group Dynamics*, 5th edn, Belmont CA, Wadsworth.

Foucault, M. (1980) *Power/Knowledge; Selected Interviews and Other Writings 1972–77*, Brighton, Harvester Press.

Fowler, M. (1996) 'The Organisation of Clinical Supervision within the Nursing Profession: A Review of the Literature', *Journal of Advanced Nursing*, 23.

Freire, P. (1972) *Pedagogy of the Oppressed*, Harmondsworth, Penguin.

Freshwater, D. (1999) 'Clinical Supervision, Reflective Practice and Guided Discovery: Clinical Supervision', *British Journal of Nursing*, 8(20).

Freshwater, D. (2000) 'Cross currents: Against Cultural Narration', *Journal of Advanced Nursing*, 32 (2).

Freshwater, D. (2004) 'Aesthetics and Evidence-Based Practice in Nursing: An Oxymoron?' *International Journal of Human Caring*, 8(2).

Freshwater, D. (2007) 'Reflective Practice and Clinical Supervision: Two Sides of the Same Coin?', in Bishop (2007).

Freshwater, D. and Avis, M. (2004) 'Analysing Interpretation and Reinterpreting Analysis: Exploring the Logic of Critical Reflection', *Nursing Philosophy*, 5.

Freshwater, D. and Rolfe, G. (2001) 'Critical Reflexivity: A Politically and Ethically Engaged Method for Nursing', *NT Research*, 6(1).

Freshwater, D. and Stickley, T. (2004) 'The Heart of the Art: Emotional Intelligence in Nurse Education', *Nursing Inquiry*, 11(2).

Freshwater, D., Taylor, B. and Sherwood, G. (2008) *International Textbook of Reflective Practice in Nursing*, Oxford, Blackwell Publishing.

Gadamer, H.-G. (1975) *Truth and Method,* New York, Continuum.

Gadamer, H.-G. (1996) *The Enigma of Health*, Cambridge, Polity Press.

REFERENCES

Garland, J.A., Jones, H.E. and Kolodny, R.L. (1965) 'A Model for Stages of Development in Social Work Groups', in Berstein (1965).

Garnham, A. and Oakhill, J. (1994) *Thinking and Reasoning*, Oxford, Blackwell.

Gibbs, G. (1988) *Learning by Doing: A Guide to Teaching and Learning Methods*, Oxford, Further Education Unit, Oxford Polytechnic.

Giddens, A. (1984) *The Constitution Of Society: Outline of a Theory of Structuration*, University of California Press, Berkeley.

Gilbert, T. (2001) 'Reflective Practice and Supervision: Meticulous Rituals of the Confessional', *Journal of Advanced Nursing*, 36(2).

Glass, N. (2000) 'Speaking Feminisms and Nursing', in Greenwood (2000).

Glaze, J.E. (2002) 'Stages in Coming to Terms with Reflection: Student Advanced Nurse Practitioners' Perceptions of their Reflective Journeys', *Journal of Advanced Nursing*, 37(3).

Gould, N. and Taylor, I. (eds) (1996) *Reflective Learning for Social Work*, Aldershot, Ashgate.

Grant, A., Kinnersley, P., Metcalf, E., Pill, R. and Houston, H. (2006) 'Students' Views of Reflective Learning Techniques: An Efficacy Study at a UK Medical School', *Medical Education*, 40.

Gray, G. and Pratt, R. (eds) (1991) *Towards a Discipline of Nursing*, Melbourne, Churchill Liningstone, Melbourne.

Greenwood, J. (ed.) (2000) *Nursing Theory in Australia: Development and Application*, Frenchs Forest, New South Wales, Pearson Education Australia.

Haber, J., Krainovich-Miller, D., McMahon, A. and Price-Hoskins, P. (1997), cited in Espeland and Shanta (2001).

Habermas, J. (1974) *Theory and Practice*, London, Heinemann.

Habermas, J. (1987) *Knowledge and Human Interest*, Cambridge, Polity Press.

Harris, M. (2008) 'Scaffolding Reflective Journal Writing – Negotiating Power, Play and Position', *Nurse Education Today*, 28.

Hawkins, P. and Shohet, R. (2006) *Supervision in the Helping Professions*, 3rd edn, Milton Keynes, Open University Press.

Heath, H. and Freshwater, D. (2000) 'Clinical Supervision as an Emancipatory Process: Avoiding Inappropriate Intent', *Journal of Advanced Nursing*, 32(5).

Heron, J. (1981) *Assessment*, Guildford, Human Potential Resource Group, University of Surrey.

Holloway, E. (1995) *Clinical Supervision. A Systems Approach*, London, Sage.

Holloway, I. and Freshwater, D. (2007) *Narrative Research in Nursing*. Oxford, Blackwell Publishing.

Holly, M. (1984) *Keeping a Personal Professional Journal*, Victoria, Deakin University Press.

Holm, A., Lantz, I. and Severinsson, E. (1998) 'Nursing Students' Experiences of the Effects of Continual Process-Oriented Group Supervision', *Journal of Nursing Management*, 6.

Holm, D. and Stephenson, S. (1994) Reflection – A Student's Perspective, in Palmer, Burns and Bulman (1994).

Jackson, D., Mannix, J., Faga, P. and Gillies, D. (2005) 'Raising Families: Urban Women's Experiences of Requiring Support', *Contemporary Nurse*, 18(1–2).

Jarvis, P., Holford, J. and Griffin, C. (1998) *The Theory and Practice of Learning*, London, Kogan Page.

Jasper, M. (1999) 'Assessing and Improving Student Outcomes through Reflective Writing,' in Rust (1999).

Jasper, M. (2005) 'Editorial. New Nursing Roles – Implications for Nursing', *Journal of Nursing Management*, 13.

Jasper, M. (2006) *Professional Development, Reflection and Decision-Making*, Oxford, Blackwell Publishing.

Jasper, M. (2008) 'Using Reflective Journals and Diaries to Enhance Practice and Learning', in Bulman and Schutz (2008).

Johns, C. (1993) 'Professional Supervision', *Journal of Nursing Management*, 1.

Johns, C. (1996) 'Visualising and Realising Caring in Practice through Guided Reflection', *Journal of Advanced Nursing*, 24(6).

Johns, C. (1998) Opening the Doors of Perception, in Johns and Freshwater (1998).

Johns, C. (2000) *Becoming a Reflective Practitioner*, Oxford, Blackwell Science.

Johns, C. (2001) 'Depending on the Intent and Emphasis of the Supervisor, Clinical Supervision can be a Different Experience,' *Journal of Nursing Management*, 9(3).

Johns, C. (2003) 'Easing into the Light', *International Journal for Human Caring*, 7(1).

Johns, C. (2004) *Becoming a Reflective Practitioner*, 2nd edn, Oxford, Blackwell Publishing.

Johns, C. (2006) *Engaging Reflection in Practice: A Narrative Approach*, Oxford, Blackwell Publishing.

Johns, C. (2009) *Becoming a Reflective Practitioner*, 3rd edn, Oxford, Wiley Blackwell.

Johns, C. and Freshwater, D. (2005) *Transforming Nursing through Reflective Practice*, 2nd edn, Oxford, Blackwell Science.

Johns, C. and McCormack, B. (1998) 'Unfolding the Conditions where the Transformative Potential of Guided Reflection (Clinical Supervision) might Flourish or Flounder', in Johns and Freshwater (1998).

Jones, A. (2003) 'Some Benefits Experienced by Hospice Nurses from Group Clinical Supervision', *European Journal of Cancer Care*, 12.

Jones, A. (2006) 'Group-Format Clinical Supervision for Hospice Nurses', *European Journal of Cancer Care*, 15.

Kim, H.S. (1999) 'Critical Reflective Inquiry for Knowledge Development in Nursing Practice', *Journal of Advanced Nursing*, 29(5).

Kingston, P. and Smith, D. (1983) 'Preparation for Live Consultation and Live Supervision when Working Without a One-Way Screen', *Journal of Family Therapy*, 5.

Kintgen Andrews, J. (1991) 'Critical Thinking and Nursing Education: Perplexities and Insights', *Journal of Nursing Education*, 30.

Knowles, M. (1984) *The Adult Learner: A Neglected Species* (3rd edn), Houston: Gulf.

Koch, T. and Harrington, A. (1998) Reconceptualizing Rigour: The Case for Reflexivity, *Journal of Advanced Nursing* 28(4).

Kohner, N. (1994) *Clinical Supervision in Practice*, London, Kings Fund Centre.

Kolb, D.A. (1984) *Experiential Learning: Experience as the Source of Learning and Development*, New Jersey, Prentice-Hall.

Kolb, D.A., Osland, J.S. and Rubin, I.M. (1995) *Organizational Behavior*, 6th edn, Englewood Cliffs, NJ, Prentice-Hall.

Kuhn, T.S. (1996) *The Structure of Scientific Revolutions*, 3rd edn, Chicago, IL, University of Chicago Press.

Lahteenmaki, M.-L. (2005) 'Reflectivity in Supervised Practice: Conventional and Transformative Approaches to Physiotherapy', *Learning in Health and Social Care*, 4(1).

Lenny, M.J. (2006) 'Inclusion, Projections of Difference and Reflective Practice: An Interactionist Perspective', *Reflective Practice*, 7(2).

Levine, B. (1991) *Group Psychotherapy, Practice and Development*, New York, Prentice-Hall.

Lindahl, B. and Norberg, A. (2002) 'Clinical Group Supervision in an Intensive Care unit', *Journal of Clinical Nursing*, 11.

Lindgren, B., Brulin, C., Holmlund, K. and Athlin, E. (2005) 'Nursing Students' Perception of Group Supervision during Clinical Training', *Journal of Clinical Nursing*, 14.

Lindsay, T. and Orton, S. (2008) *Groupwork Practice in Social Work*, Exeter, Learning Matters.

Linton, J.M. (2003) 'A Preliminary Qualitative Investigation of Group Processes in Group Supervision: Perspectives of Masters' Practicum Students', *Journal for Specialists in Group Work*, 28.

Lippitt, R. and White, R.K. (1953) 'Leader Behaviour and Member Reaction in Three Different Climates', in Cartwright and Zander (1968).

Locke, K. and Brazelton, J.K. (1997) 'Why Do We Ask Them To Write, or Whose Writing is it Anyway?', *Journal of Management Education*, 21.

Lufe, J. (1969) *Of Human Interactions. The Johari Model*, Palo Alto, Mayfield.

Lumby, J. (1997) Liver Transplantation: The Death/Life Paradox, *International Journal of Nursing Practice*, 3.

MacKeracher, D. (2004) *Making Sense of Adult Learning*, 2nd edn, Toronto, University of Toronto Press.

Mackintosh, C. (1998) 'Reflection: A Flawed Strategy for the Nursing Profession', *Nurse Education Today*, 18.

Maich, N.M., Brown, B. and Royle, J. (2000) '"Becoming" through Reflection and Professional Portfolios: The Voice of Growth in Nursing', *Reflective Practice*, 1(3).

Malinski, V. (2002) Research Issues: Nursing Research and the Human Sciences, *Nursing Science Quarterly*, 15(1).

Mantzoukas, S. and Jasper, M. (2004) 'Reflective Practice and Daily Ward Reality: A Covert Power Game', *Issues in Clinical Nursing*, 13.

Marken, M. and Payne, M. (eds) (1986) *Enabling and Ensuring*, Leicester, National Youth Bureau and Council for Education and Training in Youth and Community Work.

McGill, I. and Beaty, L. (2001) *Action Learning: A Guide for Professional, Management and Educational Development*, 2nd edn, Abingdon, Taylor Francis.

Meyers, R.G. (2006) *Understanding Empiricism*, Chesham, Acumen.

Mezirow, J. (1981) A Critical Theory of Adult Learning and Education, *Adult Education*, 32.

Milinkovic, D. and Field, N. (2005) Demystifying the Reflective Clinical Journal, *Radiography*, 11.

Montalvo, B. (1973) Aspects of Live Supervision, *Family Process*, 12.

Morgan, J., Rawlinson, M. and Weaver, M. (2006) 'Facilitating Online Reflective Learning for Health and Social Care Professionals', *Open Learning*, 21(2).

Morton-Cooper, A. and Palmer, A. (2000) *Mentoring, Preceptorship and Clinical Supervision: A Guide to Support Roles in Clinical practice*, 2nd edn, Oxford, Blackwell Science.

Newell, R. (1992) 'Anxiety, Accuracy and Reflection: The Limits of Professional Development', *Journal of Advanced Nursing*, 17.

Nichols, K. and Jenkinson, J. (2006) *Leading a Support Group: A Practical Guide*, Maidenhead, Open University Press.

NMC (Nursing & Midwifery Council) (2002) *Supporting Nurses and Midwives through Lifelong Learning*, London, Nursing & Midwifery Council.

Northcott, N. (2000) Clinical Supervision – Professional Development or Management Control?, in Spouse and Refern, 2000.

Obholzer, A. and Roberts, V.Z. (eds) (1994) *The Unconscious at Work*, London, Routledge.

Ogren, M.L. and Jonsson, C.O. (2003) 'Psychotherapeutic Skills Following Group Supervision According to Supervisees and Supervisors', *The Clinical Supervisor*, 22.

Orland-Barak, L. (2005) 'Portfolios as evidence of reflective practice, what remains "untold"', *Educational Research*, 47(1).

Page, S. and Woskett, V. (1994) *Supervising the Counsellor*, London, Routledge.

Palmer, A., Burns, S. and Bulman, C. (eds) (1994), *Reflective Practice in Nursing*, Oxford, Blackwell Science.

Pateman, B. (2000) 'Feminist Research or Humanistic Research? Experiences of Studying Prostatectomy', *Journal of Clinical Nursing*, 9(2).

Pellat, G. (2003) 'Ethnography and Reflexivity: Emotions and Feelings in Fieldwork', *Nurse Researcher*, 19(3).

Pesut, D.J. and Herman, J. (1999) *Clinical Reasoning: The Art & Science of Critical & Creative Thinking*, New York, Delmar Publishers.

Phelan, P. and Reynolds, P. (1996) *Argument and Evidence*, London, Routledge.

Phillips, J. (2001) *Groupwork in Social Care: Planning and Setting Up Groups*, London, Jessica Kingsley.

Plack, M. and Greenberg, L. (2005) 'The Reflective Practitioner: Reaching for Excellence in Practice', *Pediatrics*, 1161.

Platzer, H., Blake, D. and Ashford, D. (2000) 'Barriers to Learning from Reflection: A Study of the Use of Groupwork with Post-Registration Nurses', *Journal of Advanced Nursing* 31(5).

Plummer, K. (1983) *Documents of Life: An Introduction to the Problems and Literature of a Humanistic Method*, London, George Allen & Unwin.

Polkinghorne, D.E. (1988) *Narrative Knowing and the Human Sciences*, State University of New York, Albany.

Powers, B. and Knapp, P. (2006) *Dictionary of Nursing Theory and Research*, 3rd edn, New York, Springer.

Proctor, B. (1986) Supervision: A Co-operative Exercise in Accountability, in Marken and Payne, (1986).

Progoff, I. (1975) *At a Journal Workshop: The Basic Text and Guide for Using the Journal*, New York, Dialogue House Library.

Rai, L. (2006) 'Owning (up to) Reflective Writing in Social Work Education', *Social Work*, 25(8).

Redl, F. (1951) 'Art of Group Composition', in Schulze (1951).

Redmond, B. (2006) *Reflection-in-action: Developing Reflective Practice in Health and Social Care*, Aldershot, Ashgate Publishing.

Reece Jones, P. (1995) 'Hindsight Bias in Reflective Practice: An Empirical Investigation', *Journal of Advanced Nursing*, 21.

Reichelt, S., Gullestad, S.E., Hansen, B.R., Ronnestad, M.H., Torgersen, A.M., Jacobsen, C.H., Nielsen, G.H. and Skjerve, J. (2009) 'Nondisclosure in Psychotherapy Group Supervision: The Supervisee Perspective', *Nordic Psychology*, 61(4).

Reimers, S. and Treacher, A. (1995) *Introducing User friendly Family Therapy*, London, Routledge.

Rideout, E. (2001) *Transforming Nursing Education through Problem Based Learning*, Sudbury, Jones & Bartlett Publishers.

Ringer, T.M. (2002) *Group Action: The Dynamics of Groups in Therapeutic, Educational and Corporate Settings*, London, Jessica Kingsley.

Rogers, C. (1983) *Freedom to Learn for the 80s*, Columbus, Merrill.

Rogers, C.R. (1961) *Client Centred Therapy*, London, Constable.

Rolfe, G. (1994) 'Towards a New Model of Nursing Research', *Journal of Advanced Nursing*, 19.

Rolfe, G. (1998) *Expanding Nursing Knowledge: Understanding and Researching Your Own Practice*, Oxford, Butterworth Heinemann.

Rolfe, G. (2001) 'Reflective Practice: Where Now?', *Nurse Education in Practice*, 2.

Rolfe, G. (2003) 'Is There a Place for Reflection in the Nursing Curriculum? A Reply to Newell', *Clinical Effectiveness in Nursing*, 7(1).

Rolfe, G. (2005a) 'Editorial. Evidence-Based Practice and the Need for Conceptual Clarity', *Practice Development in Health Care*, 4(1).

Rolfe, G. (2005b) 'Response. Where is John Paley When You Need Him?' *Nursing Philosophy*, 6.

Rolfe, G. (2005c) 'The Deconstructing Angel: Nursing, Reflection and Evidence-Based Practice', *Nursing Inquiry*, 12.

Rolfe, G. and Freshwater, D. (2005) '"To save the Honour of Thinking": A Slightly Petulant Response to Griffiths,' *International Journal of Nursing Studies* 42.

Rolfe, G. and Gardner, L.D. (2006) '"Do Not Ask Who I Am...": Confession, Emancipation And (Self) Management through Reflection,' *Journal of Nursing Management*, 14.

Rolfe, G., Freshwater, D. and Jasper, M. (2001) *Critical Reflection for Nursing and the Helping Professions: A User's Guide*, Basingstoke, Palgrave Macmillan.

Rosenbaum, M., Ferguson, K., Broderick, A. (2008) Five-Year Experience: Reflective Writing in a Preclinical End-of-Life Care Curriculum, *The Permanente Journal*, 12(2).

Rust, C. (ed) (1999) *Improving Student Learning – Improving Student Learning Outcomes*, Oxford: Oxford Centre for Staff Development.

Ryle, G. (1963) *The Concept of Mind*, Harmondsworth, Penguin.

Saarikoski, M., Warne, T., Aunio, R. and Leino-Kilpi, H. (2006) 'Group Supervision in Facilitating Learning and Teaching in Mental Health Clinical Placements: A Case Example of One Student Group', *Issues in Mental Health Nursing*, 27.

Sackett, D.L., Rosenberg, W.M.C., Muir Gray, J.A., Haynes, R.B. and Scott Richardson, W. (1996) Evidence Based Medicine: What It Is and What It Isn't, *British Medical Journal*, 312.

Schön, D. (1983) *The Reflective Practitioner*, London, Temple Smith.

Schön, D. (1987) *Educating the Reflective Practitioner*, San Francisco, Jossey-Bass.

Schulze, S. (ed.) (1951) *Creative Living in a Children's Institution*, New York, Free Association Press.

Schutz, W.C. (1958) *FIRO: A Three Dimensional Theory of Interpersonal Behaviour*, New York, Holt, Rinehart & Winston.

Shapiro, J., Kasman, D. and Shafer, A. (2006) Words and Wards: A Model of Reflective Writing and Its Uses in Medical Education, *Journal of Medical Humanities*, 27.

Sharples, M. (1999) *How We Write*, London, Routledge.

Simpson, E. and Courtney, M. (2007) 'A Framework Guiding Critical Thinking through Reflective Journal Documentation: A Middle Eastern Experience', *International Journal of Nursing Practice*, 13.

Spouse, J. and Redfern, L. (2000) 'Creating a Quality Service', in Spouse and Redfern (2000b).

Spouse, J. and Redfern, L. (eds) (2000b) *Successful Supervision in Health Care Practice*, Oxford, Blackwell Science.

Stoltenberg, C.D. and Delworth, V. (1987) *Supervising Counsellors and Therapists*, San Francisco, Jossey-Bass.

Sutton, L. and Dalley, J. (2008) 'Reflection in an Intermediate Care Team', *Physiotherapy*, 94.

Swindell, M. and Watson, J. (2006) 'Teaching Ethics Through Self-Reflective Journaling', *Journal of Social Work Values and Ethics*, 3(2), accessed on June 2, 2010 from: http://www.socialworker.com/jswve/content/view/47/50/

Taylor, B. (2000) *Being Human: Ordinariness in Nursing* (adapted and reprinted), Lismore, New South Wales, Southern Cross University Press.

Taylor, B.J. (2001) 'Identifying and Transforming Dysfunctional Nurse-Nurse Relationships through Reflective Practice and Action Research', *International Journal of Nursing Practice*, 7(6).

Taylor, B.J. (2006) *Reflective Practice: A Guide for Nurses and Midwives*, 2nd edn, Buckingham, Open University Press.

Taylor B. J. (2008) 'Using Reflection as an Approach to Research,' in Freshwater, Taylor and Sherwood (2008).

Taylor, C. (2006) 'Narrating Significant Experience: Reflective Accounts and the Production of (Self) Knowledge', *British Journal of Social Work*, 36.

Taylor, B., Kermode, S. and Roberts, K. (2006) *Research in Nursing and Health Care: Evidence for Practice*, 3rd edn, Australia, Thomson.

Teekman, B. (2000) 'Exploring Reflective Thinking in Nursing Practice', *Journal of Advanced Nursing*, 31(5).

Thompson, N. (2000) *Theory and Practice in Human Services*, Buckingham, Open University Press.

Thorpe, K. and Barsky, J. (2001) 'Healing through Self-Reflection', *Journal of Advanced Nursing*, 35(5).

Todd, G. and Freshwater, D. (1999) 'Reflective Practice and Guided Discovery: Clinical Supervision', *British Journal of Nursing*, 8(20).

Treacher, A. and Carpenter, J. (1992) *Using Family Therapy*, 2nd edn, Oxford, Blackwell.

Tuckman, B. (1965) 'Developmental Sequences in Small Groups', *Psychological Bulletin*, 63.

Tuttle, L. and Seibold, C. (2002) 'Ethical Issues Arising when Planning and Commencing a Research Study with Chemically Dependent Pregnant Women', *Australian Journal of Advanced Nursing*, 20(4).

UKCC (United Kingdom Central Council for Nursing, Midwifery and Health Visiting) (1996) *Position Statement on Clinical Supervision for Nursing and Health Visiting*, London, UKCC.

Usher, R. and Bryant, I. (1989) *Adult Education as Theory, Practice and Research*, London, Routledge.

Van Ments, M. (1999) *The Effective Use of Role-play*, 2nd edn, London, Kogan Page.

Van Ments, M. and Hearnden, K. (1985) *Effective Use of Games and Simulation*, Loughborough, SAGSET.

Van Ooijen, E. (2000) *Clinical Supervision: A Practical Guide*, Edinburgh, Churchill Livingstone.

Van Ooijen, E. (2003) *Clinical Supervision Made Easy*, Edinburgh, Churchill Livingstone.

Waldman, J. (2005) 'Using Evaluation Research to Support Practitioners and Service Users in Undertaking Reflective Writing for Public Dissemination', *British Journal of Social Work*, 35.

Walsh-Bowers, R. (2002) 'Constructing Qualitative Knowledge in Psychology. Students and Faculty Negotiate the Social Context of Inquiry', *Canadian Psychology*, 43(4).

Wellard, S.J. and Bethune, E. (1996) 'Reflective Journal Writing in nurse Education: Whose Interests Does it Serve?', *Journal of Advanced Nursing*, 24(5).

Whitehead, L. (2004) 'Enhancing the Quality of Hermeneutic Research: Decision Trail', *Journal of Advanced Nursing*, 45(5).

Winnicott, D.W. (1971) *Therapeutic Consultations in Child Psychiatry*, London, Hogarth Press.

Winship, G. and Hardy, S. (1999) 'Disentangling Dynamics: Group Sensitivity and Supervision', *Journal of Psychiatric and Mental Health Nursing*, 6.

Wright, H. (1989) *Group Work: Perspectives and Practice*, Harrow, Scutari Press.

Wyllie, A. (1993) 'On the Road to Discovery: A Study of the Composing Strategies of Academic Writers using the Word processor', unpublished MA thesis, University of Lancaster, cited in M. Sharples (1999), *How We Write*, London, Routledge.

Yalom, I.D. and Leszcz, M. (2005) *The Theory and Practice of Group Psychotherapy*, 5th edn, New York, Basic Books.

Index